TECHNICALLY SPEAKING

WHY ALL AMERICANS NEED TO KNOW MORE ABOUT TECHNOLOGY

Committee on Technological Literacy

National Academy of Engineering
National Research Council

Greg Pearson and A. Thomas Young, *Editors*

NATIONAL ACADEMY PRESS
Washington, D.C.

NATIONAL ACADEMY PRESS • **2101 Constitution Avenue, N.W.** • **Washington, D.C. 20418**

NOTICE: The project that is the subject of this report was approved by the Governing Board of the National Research Council, whose members are drawn from the councils of the National Academy of Sciences, the National Academy of Engineering, and the Institute of Medicine. The members of the committee responsible for the report were chosen for their special competences and with regard for appropriate balance.

This study was supported by Grant No. ESI-9814135 between the National Academy of Sciences and the National Science Foundation. Additional support for the project was provided by Battelle Memorial Institute. Any opinions, findings, conclusions, or recommendations expressed in this publication are those of the author(s) and do not necessarily reflect the views of the organizations or agencies that provided support for the project.

Library of Congress Cataloging-in-Publication Data

Technically speaking : why all Americans need to know more about
technology / Greg Pearson and A. Thomas Young, editors.
        p. cm.
Includes index.
 ISBN 0-309-08262-5
 1. Technology—Study and teaching—United States. I. Pearson, Greg.
II. Young, A. Thomas. III. National Research Council (U.S.)
 T73 .T37 2002
 607.1'073—dc21

                              2001008623

Copies of this report are available from National Academy Press, 2101 Constitution Avenue, N.W., Lockbox 285, Washington, D.C. 20055; (800) 624-6242 or (202) 334-3313 (in the Washington metropolitan area); Internet, http://www.nap.edu

Printed in the United States of America

Copyright 2002 by the National Academy of Sciences. All rights reserved.

THE NATIONAL ACADEMIES

National Academy of Sciences
National Academy of Engineering
Institute of Medicine
National Research Council

The **National Academy of Sciences** is a private, nonprofit, self-perpetuating society of distinguished scholars engaged in scientific and engineering research, dedicated to the furtherance of science and technology and to their use for the general welfare. Upon the authority of the charter granted to it by the Congress in 1863, the Academy has a mandate that requires it to advise the federal government on scientific and technical matters. Dr. Bruce M. Alberts is president of the National Academy of Sciences.

The **National Academy of Engineering** was established in 1964, under the charter of the National Academy of Sciences, as a parallel organization of outstanding engineers. It is autonomous in its administration and in the selection of its members, sharing with the National Academy of Sciences the responsibility for advising the federal government. The National Academy of Engineering also sponsors engineering programs aimed at meeting national needs, encourages education and research, and recognizes the superior achievements of engineers. Dr. Wm. A. Wulf is president of the National Academy of Engineering.

The **Institute of Medicine** was established in 1970 by the National Academy of Sciences to secure the services of eminent members of appropriate professions in the examination of policy matters pertaining to the health of the public. The Institute acts under the responsibility given to the National Academy of Sciences by its congressional charter to be an adviser to the federal government and, upon its own initiative, to identify issues of medical care, research, and education. Dr. Kenneth I. Shine is president of the Institute of Medicine.

The **National Research Council** was organized by the National Academy of Sciences in 1916 to associate the broad community of science and technology with the Academy's purposes of furthering knowledge and advising the federal government. Functioning in accordance with general policies determined by the Academy, the Council has become the principal operating agency of both the National Academy of Sciences and the National Academy of Engineering in providing services to the government, the public, and the scientific and engineering communities. The Council is administered jointly by both Academies and the Institute of Medicine. Dr. Bruce M. Alberts and Dr. Wm. A. Wulf are chairman and vice chairman, respectively, of the National Research Council.

Committee on Technological Literacy

A. THOMAS YOUNG, *Chair*, Lockheed Martin Corporation (retired), North Potomac, Maryland
PAUL ALLAN, Pacific Science Center, Seattle, Washington
WILLIAM ANDERS, General Dynamics Co. (retired), Deer Harbor, Washington
TAFT H. BROOME, JR., Howard University, Washington, D.C.
JONATHAN R. COLE, Columbia University, New York, New York
RODNEY L. CUSTER, Illinois State University, Normal, Illinois
GOÉRY DELACÔTE, The Exploratorium, San Francisco, California
DENICE DENTON, University of Washington, Seattle
PAUL DE VORE, PWD Associates, Morgantown, West Virginia
KAREN FALKENBERG, Emory University, Atlanta, Georgia
SHELAGH A. GALLAGHER, University of North Carolina, Charlotte
JOYCE GARDELLA, Gardella & Associates, Watertown, Massachusetts
DAVID T. HARRISON, Seminole Community College, Sanford, Florida
PAUL HOFFMAN, Writer and Consultant, Woodstock, New York
JONDEL (J.D.) HOYE, Keep the Change, Inc., Aptos, California
THOMAS P. HUGHES, University of Pennsylvania, Philadelphia
MAE JEMISON, Jemison Group, Inc., Houston, Texas
F. JAMES RUTHERFORD, American Association for the Advancement of Science, Washington, D.C.
KATHRYN C. THORNTON, University of Virginia, Charlottesville
ROBERT TINKER, Concord Consortium, Concord, Massachusetts

Project Staff

GREG PEARSON, Study Director and Program Officer, National Academy of Engineering (NAE)
JAY LABOV, Deputy Director, Center for Education, National Research Council
KATHARINE GRAMLING, Research Assistant, NAE (September 2000 to project end)
MATTHEW CAIA, Senior Project Assistant, NAE (June 2001 to project end)

MARK LORIE, Project Assistant, NAE (April 1999 to August 2000)
CAROL R. ARENBERG, Managing Editor, NAE
ROBERT POOL, Freelance Writer

Preface

This report and a companion website (www.nae.edu/techlit) are the final products of a two-year study by the Committee on Technological Literacy, a group of experts on diverse subjects under the auspices of the National Academy of Engineering (NAE) and the Center for Education, part of the National Research Council (NRC). The committee's charge was to begin to develop among relevant communities a common understanding of what technological literacy is, how important it is to the nation, and how it can be achieved. The charge reflects the interests and goals of the two project sponsors, the National Science Foundation (NSF) and Battelle Memorial Institute, as well as the priorities of the National Academies.

NAE President Bill Wulf, who has championed the cause of technological literacy throughout his tenure at the Academies, contributed greatly to the success of the project. The idea for the study arose from his strong interests in improving both K-12 education and the public understanding of engineering and technology. In the mid-1990s, Dr. Wulf initiated discussions among staff at the NAE, NRC, NSF, and other groups on this issue. The discussions revealed that the concept of technological literacy is poorly understood and significantly undervalued.

The committee adopted a broad definition of technology that encompasses both the tangible artifacts of the human-designed world (e.g., bridges, automobiles, computers, satellites, medical imaging devices, drugs, genetically engineered plants) and the systems of which these artifacts are a part (e.g., transportation, communications, health care, food production), as well as the people, infrastructure, and processes required to design, manufacture, operate, and repair the artifacts. This comprehensive view of technology differs considerably from the more common, narrower public conception, which associates technology almost exclusively with computers and other electronics.

The report is intended for a very broad audience, including schools of education, schools of engineering, K-12 teachers and teacher organizations, developers of curriculum and instructional materials, federal and state policy makers, industry and nonindustry supporters of education reform, and science and technology centers and museums. Most of the committee's recommendations are directed toward these groups, which are particularly well positioned to have a positive influence on the development of technological literacy.

The committee met six times and sponsored two workshops. At the first workshop, in September 1999, a framework was developed based on the issues of education, the workforce, and democracy to guide the committee's thinking in subsequent stages. At the second workshop, in March 2000, the program was focused on national and international activities that have contributed to the development of technological literacy. The committee's deliberations were based on the results of these workshops and a survey of the relevant literature by project staff. The final document also reflects the personal and professional experience and judgment of committee members. The report was released publicly at a symposium held at the National Academies in January 2002.

The idea that all Americans should be better prepared to navigate our highly technological world has been advocated by many individuals and groups for years. Nevertheless, the issue of technological literacy is virtually invisible on the national agenda. This is especially disturbing in a time when technology is a dominant force in society. By presenting the topic in a straightforward and compelling manner, the committee hopes technological literacy will be put "on the map" and the way will be cleared for a meaningful movement toward technological literacy in the United States.

A. Thomas Young
Chair
Committee on Technological Literacy

Acknowledgments

This report has been reviewed in draft form by individuals chosen for their diverse perspectives and technical expertise, in accordance with procedures approved by the NRC's Report Review Committee. The purpose of this independent review is to provide candid and critical comments that will assist the institution in making its published report as sound as possible and to ensure that the report meets institutional standards for objectivity, evidence, and responsiveness to the study charge. The review comments and draft manuscript remain confidential to protect the integrity of the deliberative process. We wish to thank the following individuals for their review of this report:

Alice M. Agogino, University of California, Berkeley
Arden L. Bement, Purdue University
Daniel M. Hull, Center for Occupational Research and
    Development
Patricia Hutchinson, The College of New Jersey
Peter Joyce, Cisco Systems, Inc.
Shirley M. McBay, Quality Education for Minorities Network
Henry Petroski, Duke University
Robert Semper, San Francisco Exploratorium
Kendall Starkweather, International Technology Education
    Association
Robert Yager, University of Iowa Science Education Center

Although the reviewers listed above have provided many constructive comments and suggestions, they were not asked to endorse the conclusions or recommendations nor did they see the final draft of the report before its release. The review of this report was overseen by Mildred S. Dresselhaus, Massachusetts Institute of Technology, and Elsa M. Garmire, Dartmouth College. Appointed by the National Research Council, they were responsible for making certain that an independent examination of this report was carried out in accordance with institutional procedures and that all review comments were carefully considered. Responsibility for the final content of this report rests entirely with the authoring committee and the institution.

In addition to the reviewers, many individuals and organizations assisted in the development of this report. Rodger Bybee played a central role in the conception of this project during the time he headed NRC activities related to science and mathematics education, and he contributed to its success after he left the institution. Kendall Starkweather, Bill Dugger, and Pam Newberry, all at the International Technology Education Association, provided information and support throughout the project. Dennis Cheek, at the Rhode Island Department of Education, conducted extensive research on behalf of the committee. John Staudenmaier, at Boston College, prepared a key background paper that helped put the committee's charge in context. Writer Robert Pool, who crafted several key sections of the report, successfully captured the essence of the committee's sometimes wide-ranging discussions. The project's outside evaluators, Jill Russell and Neal Grandgenett, provided useful and timely suggestions, which improved the quality of the final product. The participants in the committee's two workshops provided an invaluable stimulus to the committee's deliberations.

Finally, no project of this scope is possible without the support of staff. The committee was fortunate to have the assistance of a very capable group. Our thanks go to Mark Lorie and Matthew Caia, who performed countless tasks, from conducting research to handling the logistics of committee meetings and workshops. Katharine Gramling served in a variety of capacities, including designing and overseeing the construction of the project website. Thanks are also due to NAE editor Carol R. Arenberg, who substantially improved the report's readability. Special recognition goes to the staff leaders of the project, Jay Labov at the NRC Center for Education, and, especially, Greg Pearson at the NAE, whose patience and behind-the-scenes work made the committee's work not only possible but pleasurable.

Contents

TECHNICALLY SPEAKING

Executive Summary

At the heart of our modern technological society lies an unacknowledged paradox. Although the United States is increasingly defined by and dependent on technology and is adopting new technologies at a breathtaking pace, its citizens are not equipped to make well-considered decisions or to think critically about technology. As a society, we are not even fully aware of or conversant with the technologies we use every day. In short, we are not "technologically literate."

Technology has become so user friendly it is largely "invisible." Americans use technology with a minimal comprehension of how or why it works or the implications of its use or even where it comes from. We drive high-tech cars but know little more than how to operate the steering wheel, gas pedal, and brake pedal. We fill shopping carts with highly processed foods but are largely ignorant of their content, or how they are developed, grown, packaged, or delivered. We click on a mouse and transmit data over thousands of miles without understanding how this is possible or who might have access to the information.

Available evidence shows that American adults and children have a poor understanding of the essential characteristics of technology, how it influences society, and how people can and do affect its development. Neither the educational system nor the policy-making apparatus in the United States has recognized the importance of technological literacy.

Thus the paradox: Even as technology has become increasingly important in our lives, it has receded from view. Americans are poorly equipped to recognize, let alone ponder or address, the challenges technology poses or the problems it could solve. And the mismatch is growing. Although our use of technology is increasing apace, there is no sign of a corresponding improvement in our ability to deal with issues relating to technology.

To take full advantage of the benefits and to recognize, address, or even avoid some of the pitfalls of technology, we must become better stewards of technological change. Unfortunately, we are ill prepared to meet this goal. This report represents a mandate—an urgent call—for technological literacy in the United States.

The Report

This report and a companion website (<www.nae.edu/techlit>) are the final products of a two-year study by the Committee on Technological Literacy, a group of experts from diverse fields operating under the auspices of the National Academy of Engineering (NAE) and the National Research Council (NRC) Center for Education. The committee was charged with developing a vision for technological literacy in the United States and recommending ways for achieving that vision. The project was funded by the National Science Foundation (NSF) and Battelle Memorial Institute.

The report is directed at groups that are well positioned to influence the development of technological literacy, including schools of education, schools of engineering, K-12 teachers and teacher organizations, developers of curriculum and instructional materials, federal and state policy makers, industry and nonindustry supporters of educational reform, and science and technology centers and museums.

What Is Technology?

In its broadest sense, technology is the process by which humans modify nature to meet their needs and wants. However, most people think of technology only in terms of its artifacts: computers and software, aircraft, pesticides, water-treatment plants, birth-control pills, and microwave ovens, to name a few. But technology is more than its tangible products. An equally important aspect of technology is the knowledge and processes necessary to create and operate those products, such as engineering know-how and design, manufacturing expertise, various technical skills, and so on. Technology also includes all of the infrastructure

> **Technology comprises the entire system of people and organizations, knowledge, processes, and devices that go into creating and operating technological artifacts, as well as the artifacts themselves.**

necessary for the design, manufacture, operation, and repair of technological artifacts, from corporate headquarters and engineering schools to manufacturing plants and maintenance facilities.

What Is Technological Literacy?

Technological literacy encompasses three interdependent dimensions—knowledge, ways of thinking and acting, and capabilities (Box ES-1). Like literacy in reading, mathematics, science, or history, the goal of technological literacy is to provide people with the tools to participate intelligently and thoughtfully in the world around them. The kinds of things a technologically literate person must know can vary from society to society and from era to era.

Benefits of Technological Literacy

Individuals and the country as a whole would benefit greatly from a higher level of technological literacy. For one thing, people at all levels of society would be better prepared to make well-informed decisions on matters that affect, or are affected by, technology. For example, consumers must routinely decide whether or not to use particular products and how to use them. Technologically literate consumers would be able to make more critical assessments of technologies and, therefore, more informed decisions.

As citizens in a democratic society, individuals are also asked to help make technological choices for the country as a whole or for some part of it. Should drilling for oil be allowed in an environmentally sensitive area? Should the local government be allowed to install surveillance cameras in high-crime areas? Technological literacy would not determine an individual's opinion but would ensure that it would be well informed.

Technological literacy is especially important for leaders in business, government, and the media, who make or influence decisions that

> **BOX ES-1 Characteristics of a Technologically Literate Citizen**
>
> **Knowledge**
> - Recognizes the pervasiveness of technology in everyday life.
> - Understands basic engineering concepts and terms, such as systems, constraints, and trade-offs.
> - Is familiar with the nature and limitations of the engineering design process.
> - Knows some of the ways technology shapes human history and people shape technology.
> - Knows that all technologies entail risk, some that can be anticipated and some that cannot.
> - Appreciates that the development and use of technology involve trade-offs and a balance of costs and benefits.
> - Understands that technology reflects the values and culture of society.
>
> **Ways of Thinking and Acting**
> - Asks pertinent questions, of self and others, regarding the benefits and risks of technologies.
> - Seeks information about new technologies.
> - Participates, when appropriate, in decisions about the development and use of technology.
>
> **Capabilities**
> - Has a range of hands-on skills, such as using a computer for word processing and surfing the Internet and operating a variety of home and office appliances.
> - Can identify and fix simple mechanical or technological problems at home or work.
> - Can apply basic mathematical concepts related to probability, scale, and estimation to make informed judgments about technological risks and benefits.

affect many others, sometimes the entire nation. These leaders would benefit from a comprehensive understanding of the nature of technology—a recognition, for example, that all technology involves trade-offs and can result in unintended consequences.

From a philosophical point of view, democratic principles imply that decisions affecting many people or the entire society should be made with as much public involvement as possible. As people gain confidence in their ability to ask questions and think critically about technological developments, they are likely to participate more in making decisions. Increased citizen participation would add legitimacy to decisions about technology and make it more likely that the public would accept those decisions. Citizen participation would also give policy makers and technical experts a better understanding of citizens' hopes and fears about technology.

Because our economy is increasingly being driven by technological innovation and because an increasing percentage of jobs require technological skills, a rise in technological literacy would have economic impacts. For example, a technologically literate public would generate a

> Democratic principles imply that decisions affecting many people or the entire society should be made with as much public involvement as possible.

more abundant supply of technologically savvy workers who would be more likely to have the knowledge and abilities—and find it easier to learn the skills they need—for jobs in today's technology-oriented workplaces. To the extent the study of technology encourages students to pursue scientific or technical careers, then improving our technological literacy would also lessen our dependence on foreign workers to fill jobs in many sectors.

Context for Technological Literacy

Most people have very few direct, hands-on connections to technology, except as finished consumer goods. They do not build the devices they use, tinker with them to improve their performance, or repair them when they break. Because of this lack of engagement, people today learn relatively little about technologies through direct experience. Thus they rarely develop the kind of practical, intuitive feel for technology that marked the relationships between earlier generations and their technologies.

The lack of familiarity with technology has given rise to a number of misconceptions. For example, most people think that technology is little more than the application of science to solve practical problems. They are not aware that modern technology is the fruit of a complex interplay between science, engineering, politics, ethics, law, and other factors. People who operate under this misconception have a limited ability to think critically about technology—to guide the development and use of a technology to ensure that it provides the greatest benefit for the greatest number of citizens. Another common misconception is that technology is either all good or all bad rather than what people and society make it. They misunderstand that the purpose for which we use a technology may be good or bad, but not the technology itself. Realistically, every technology will be more advantageous for some people, animals, plants, generations, or purposes than for others.

Because few people today have direct, hands-on experience with technology, technological literacy depends largely on what they learn in the classroom, particularly in elementary and secondary school. Unfortunately, only a small group of technology educators is involved in setting standards and developing curricula to promote technological literacy. In general, with the exception of the use of computers and the Internet, which has been strongly promoted by federal and state governments, technology is not treated seriously as a subject in grades K-12.

Even in this area, however, the focus has been on using these technologies to improve education rather than on educating students *about* technology. As a result, many K-12 educators identify technology almost exclusively with computers and related devices and so believe, erroneously, that their institutions already teach about technology.

We have almost no reliable data about the level of technological literacy among American children. Given the relatively poor showing of U.S. students on international tests in science and math, however, and given that many other Western countries teach more about technology than we do, it seems logical to assume that American students are not as technologically literate as their international counterparts. A recent Gallup poll and other data on the adult population reveal that adults are very interested in but relatively poorly informed about technology.

For the most part, policy makers at the federal and state levels have paid little or no attention to technology education or technological literacy, despite the fact that Congress and state legislatures often find themselves grappling with policy issues that require an understanding of technology. There is no evidence to suggest that legislators or their staffs are any more technologically literate than the general public.

For reasons that are at once historical, institutional, and reflective of the nature of modern technology, Americans appear to be unprepared to engage effectively and responsibly with technological change. In short, as a nation we do not appreciate the value of technological literacy and, hence, have not achieved it.

Foundation for Technological Literacy

A variety of efforts have been undertaken to increase technological literacy in the United States. In general, however, these have been small-scale projects, especially compared with efforts to boost scientific literacy and math skills. Nevertheless, past initiatives represent a resource upon which more ambitious efforts can draw.

The natural place to begin is in grades K-12, when all students could be guaranteed a basic familiarity with technology and could be encouraged to think critically about technological issues. The federal government, mainly the NSF, has funded the development of a variety of

> With the exception of the use of computers and the Internet, technology is not treated seriously as a subject in grades K-12.

technology-related curricula and instructional materials. Teachers who specialize in technology, still relatively few in number, will be essential to a serious effort to boost technological literacy. Their professional organization, the International Technology Education Association, recently published *Standards for Technological Literacy: Content for the Study of Technology*, a comprehensive statement of what students must learn in order to be technologically literate.

Courses spanning K-12 and two-year community colleges intended to prepare students for technical careers can also help develop technological literacy. Although technical competency is not the same as technological literacy, the development of skills in technology can lead to a better understanding of the underlying technology and could be used as the basis for teaching about the nature, history, and role of technology in our lives. Recently, the federal government has paid more attention to technician-preparation and school-to-career programs, as well as traditional vocational education.

College and universities offer a number of options for more advanced study of technology. There are about 100 science, technology, and society programs on U.S. campuses that offer both undergraduate and graduate courses, and a number of universities have programs in the history, philosophy, or sociology of technology. Many engineering schools require that students take at least one course in the social impacts of technology.

For the adult population already out of school, the informal education system—museums and science centers, as well as television, radio, newspapers, magazines, and other media—offers opportunities for learning about and becoming engaged in a variety of issues related to technology. Some federal agencies require public input into the planning of certain types of projects, and participation in decision making can also boost technological literacy. In addition, independent organizations called community-based research groups initiate various research projects, many involving technological issues.

A sampling of print and online resources related to technological literacy appears in the appendix to the full report. This "toolkit" will be useful not only to educators and policy makers but also members of the public who wish to learn more about the subject.

> For the adult population already out of school, the informal education system offers opportunities for learning about and becoming engaged in a variety of issues related to technology.

Recommendations

The Committee on Technological Literacy reviewed direct and indirect evidence and drew on the experience and expert opinion of committee members to develop its recommendations. The committee considered the role of technology in society and our relationship to it, the ways current social, political, and educational environments affect technological literacy, and the benefits—to individuals and society at large—of greater technological literacy. The committee also reviewed initiatives—past and present—that might be a basis for a serious, sustained campaign for technological literacy. The recommendations address four areas: (1) formal and informal education; (2) research; (3) decision making; and (4) teaching excellence and educational innovation. A rationale for the recommendations and an explanation of how each could be carried out can be found in the full report.

The categories are listed in order of importance, but the recommendations relate to and support one another and should be considered as an integrated whole. For instance, the availability of better data about technological literacy and how people learn about technology will inform activities in the education sector. Initiatives to improve technological decision making are also likely to increase public sensitivity to the value of informed debate about technology. This, in turn, should boost support for research and educational reforms related to technological literacy.

Strengthening the Presence of Technology in Formal and Informal Education

Recommendation 1 Federal and state agencies that help set education policy should encourage the integration of technology content into K-12 standards, curricula, instructional materials, and student assessments in nontechnology subject areas.

Recommendation 2 The states should better align their K-12 standards, curriculum frameworks, and student assessment in the sciences, mathematics, history, social studies, civics, the arts, and language arts with national educational standards that stress the connections between these subjects and technology. National Science Foundation (NSF)- and Department of Education (DoEd)-

funded instructional materials and informal-education initiatives should also stress these connections.

Recommendation 3 NSF, DoEd, state boards of education, and others involved in K-12 science education should introduce, where appropriate, the word "technology" into the titles and contents of science standards, curricula, and instructional materials.

Recommendation 4 NSF, DoEd, and teacher education accrediting bodies should provide incentives for institutions of higher education to transform the preparation of all teachers to better equip them to teach about technology throughout the curriculum.

Developing the Research Base

Recommendation 5 The National Science Foundation should support the development of one or more assessment tools for monitoring the state of technological literacy among students and the public in the United States.

Recommendation 6 The National Science Foundation and the Department of Education should fund research on how people learn about technology, and the results should be applied in formal and informal education settings.

Enhancing Informed Decision Making

Recommendation 7 Industry, federal agencies responsible for carrying out infrastructure projects, and science and technology museums should provide more opportunities for the nontechnical public to become involved in discussions about technological developments.

Recommendation 8 Federal and state government agencies with a role in guiding or supporting the nation's scientific and technological enterprise, and private foundations concerned about good governance, should support executive education programs intended to increase the technological literacy of government and industry leaders.

Recommendation 9 U.S. engineering societies should underwrite the costs of establishing government- and media-fellow programs with the goal of creating a cadre of policy experts and journalists with a background in engineering.

Rewarding Teaching Excellence and Educational Innovation

Recommendation 10 The National Science Foundation, in collaboration with industry partners, should provide funding for awards for innovative, effective approaches to improving the technological literacy of students or the public at large.

Recommendation 11 The White House should add a Presidential Award for Excellence in Technology Teaching to those that it currently offers for mathematics and science teaching.

A Final Word

Technically Speaking: Why All Americans Need to Know More About Technology should help inform the public—especially the portion of the public that can affect policy—of the urgent need for technological literacy. But this report and its recommendations are only a starting point. The case for technological literacy must be made consistently and on an ongoing basis. As citizens gradually become more sophisticated about technological issues, they will be more willing to support measures in the schools and in the informal education arena to raise the technological literacy level of the next generation. In time, leaders in government, academia, and business will become cognizant of the importance of technological literacy to their own well-being and the welfare of the nation. Achieving this goal promises to be a slow and challenging journey but one unquestionably worth embarking on.

1
Mandate for Technological Literacy

I know of no safe depository of the ultimate powers of the society but the people themselves; and if we think them not enlightened enough to exercise their control with a wholesome discretion, the remedy is not to take it from them, but to inform their discretion by education. This is the true corrective of abuses of constitutional power.

Thomas Jefferson
letter to William C. Jarvis, September 28, 1820

Knowledge will forever govern ignorance; and a people who mean to be their own governors must arm themselves with the power which knowledge gives.

James Madison
letter to W.T. Barry, August 4, 1822

The United States is experiencing a whirlwind of technological change. Most Americans feel the change instinctively each time they encounter a new consumer gadget, read about the possibility of human cloning, or observe children as young as six or seven socializing with their school friends via online instant messaging. There have been periods, such as the late 1800s, when new inventions appeared in society at a comparable rate. But the pace of change today, with its social, economic, and other impacts, is as significant and far reaching as at any other time in history.

This report argues that "technological literacy"—an understanding of the nature and history of technology, a basic hands-on capability related to technology, and an ability to think critically about technological development—is essential for people living in a modern nation like the United States.

The argument for technological literacy is fundamentally about providing citizens with the tools to participate fully and confidently in the world around them. This aim is not unique to technological literacy; many other literacy campaigns—in reading, mathematics, science, and history, to name just a few—have similar goals. The unique aspect of this campaign is that it will prepare people—from policy makers to ordinary citizens—to make thoughtful decisions on issues that affect, or are affected by, technology. There are few things we do, or can do, today that are not influenced by technology.

This report and a companion website (<www.nae.edu/techlit>) are the products of a two-year study by the Committee on Technological Literacy, a group of diverse experts operating under the auspices of the National Academy of Engineering (NAE) and the Center for Education of the National Research Council (NRC). The committee's charge was to develop a vision for technological literacy in the United States and recommend how that vision might be achieved. The charge reflects the interests and goals of the project's sponsors, the National Science Foundation (NSF) and Battelle Memorial Institute, as well as the priorities of the National Academies.

The intended audience for the report includes schools of education, schools of engineering, K-12 teachers and teacher organizations, developers of curricula and instructional materials, federal and state policy makers, industry and nonindustry supporters of educational reform, and science and technology centers and museums. These groups are well positioned to influence the development of technological literacy.

As far into the future as our imaginations can take us, we will face challenges that depend on the development and application of technology. Better health, more abundant food, more humane living and working conditions, cleaner air and water, more effective education, and scores of other improvements in the human condition are within our grasp. But none of these improvements is guaranteed, and many problems will arise that we cannot predict. To take full advantage of the benefits and to recognize, address, or even avoid the pitfalls of technology, Americans must become better stewards of technological change. Present circumstances suggest that we are ill prepared to meet that goal. This report

Americans must become better stewards of technological change.

represents a mandate—an urgent call—for technological literacy in the United States.

What Is Technology?

In the broadest sense, technology is the process by which humans modify nature to meet their needs and wants. Most people, however, think of technology in terms of its artifacts: computers and software, aircraft, pesticides, water-treatment plants, birth-control pills, and microwave ovens, to name a few. But technology is more than these tangible products. The knowledge and processes used to create and to operate the artifacts—engineering know-how, manufacturing expertise, various technical skills, and so on—are equally important. An especially important area of knowledge is the engineering design process, of starting with a set of criteria and constraints and working toward a solution—a device, say, or a process—that meets those conditions. Engineers generate designs and then test, refine, or discard them until they find an acceptable solution. Technology also includes all of the infrastructure necessary for the design, manufacture, operation, and repair of technological artifacts, from corporate headquarters and engineering schools to manufacturing plants and maintenance facilities.

Technology comprises the entire system of people and organizations, knowledge, processes, and devices that go into creating and operating technological artifacts, as well as the artifacts themselves.

Source: Adapted from Mitchem, 1994.

Technology is a product of engineering and science, the study of the natural world. Science has two parts: (1) a body of knowledge that has been accumulated over time and (2) a process—scientific inquiry—that generates knowledge about the natural world. Engineering, too, consists of a body of knowledge—in this case knowledge of the design and creation of human-made products—and a process for solving problems.

Science and technology are tightly coupled. A scientific understanding of the natural world is the basis for much of technological development today. The design of computer chips, for instance, depends on a detailed understanding of the electrical properties of silicon and other materials. The design of a drug to fight a specific disease is made possible by knowledge of how proteins and other biological molecules are structured and interact.

Conversely, technology is the basis for a good part of scientific research. The climate models meteorologists use to study global warming require supercomputers to run the simulations. And like most of us, scientists in all fields depend on the telephone, the Internet, and jet travel.

It is difficult, if not impossible, to separate the achievements of technology from those of science. When the Apollo 11 spacecraft put Neil Armstrong and Buzz Aldrin on the moon, many people called it a victory of science. When a new type of material, such as lightweight, superstrong composites, emerges on the market, newspapers often report it as a scientific advance. Genetic engineering of crops to resist insects is also usually attributed wholly to science. And although science is integral to all of these advances, they are also examples of technology, the application of unique skills, knowledge, and techniques, which is quite different from science.

Technology is also closely associated with innovation, the transformation of ideas into new and useful products or processes. Innovation requires not only creative people and organizations, but also the availability of technology and science and engineering talent. Technology and innovation are synergistic. The development of gene-sequencing machines, for example, has made the decoding of the human genome possible, and that knowledge is fueling a revolution in diagnostic, therapeutic, and other biomedical innovations.

Technological Literacy

Technological literacy encompasses at least three distinct dimensions: knowledge, ways of thinking and acting, and capabilities.

Over the years, many individuals and organizations have attempted to describe the essential elements of technological literacy (AAAS, 1990a, 1993; Dyrenfurth, 1991; ITEA, 2000). In one popular conception, technological literacy is equated with a facility with computers (Fanning, 2001; 21st Century Workforce Commission, 2000). This conception is prevalent in the U.S. educational sector, where considerable efforts and resources have been invested in making educational technol-

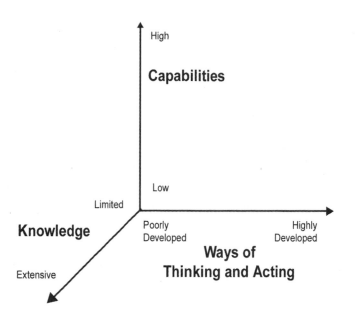

FIGURE 1-1   The dimensions of technological literacy.

ogy, much of it computer related, more available and useful (e.g., U.S. Department of Education, 1996).

Although computer skills are an important aspect of being an educated, well-rounded citizen in a modern country like the United States, the conception of technological literacy used in this report is much broader and more complex. It encompasses three interdependent dimensions: (1) knowledge; (2) ways of thinking and acting;[1] and (3) capabilities (Figure 1-1).

In practice, it is impossible to separate the dimensions from one another. It is hard to imagine a person with technological capability who does not also know something about the workings of technology, or a person who can think critically about a technological issue who does not also have some conceptual or factual knowledge of technology and science. So, although such a framework can be helpful in thinking and talking about technological literacy, it is important to remember the dimensions are arbitrary divisions.

The dimensions of technological literacy can be placed along a

---

[1]The phrase "ways of thinking and acting" is adapted from the American Association for the Advancement of Science's Project 2061, which used the term to describe the critical thinking skills (also called "habits of mind") essential to science literacy (AAAS, 1990b).

continuum—from low to high, poorly developed to well developed, limited to extensive. Every technologically literate individual has a unique combination of knowledge, ways of thinking and acting, and capabilities. In addition, an individual's locus along any dimension changes over time with education and life experience. Different job and life circumstances require different levels and types of literacy. For example, a state legislator involved in a debate about the merits of constructing new power plants to meet future electricity demand ought to understand at a fairly sophisticated level the technological concepts of trade-offs, constraints, and systems. He or she must also understand enough details about power generation to sort through conflicting claims by utility companies, environmental lobbyists, and other stakeholder groups. The average consumer pondering the purchase of a new high-definition television may be well served by a more basic understanding of the technology—for example, the differences between digital and analog signals—and a smaller set of critical thinking skills.

> **Different job and life circumstances require different levels and types of literacy.**

One useful way to think about technological literacy is as a component of the more general, or "cultural," literacy popularized by E.D. Hirsch, Jr. Hirsch (1988) pointed out that literate people in every society and every culture share a body of knowledge that enables them to communicate with each other and make sense of the world around them. The kinds of things a literate person knows will vary from society to society and from era to era; so there is no absolute definition of literacy. In the early twenty-first century, however, cultural literacy must have a large technological component.

The importance of technological literacy to individuals living in a modern society is not a new idea. Almost 20 years ago, for example, advisors to the National Science Board called for increased technological literacy (CPEMST, 1983):

> We must return to the basics, but the "basics" of the 21st century are not only reading, writing, and arithmetic. They include communication and higher problem-solving skills, and scientific and technological literacy—the thinking tools that allow us to understand the technological world around us.

As we begin the twenty-first century, the need for increasing technological literacy has become even greater, first because the influence of technology over people's lives has increased dramatically and second because, as a society, we have not put a high priority on technological literacy.

A Technologically Literate Person

Although there is no archetype of a technologically literate person, we can describe some general characteristics such a person ought to possess (Box 1-1). A technologically literate person should be able to recognize technology in its many forms, and should understand that the line between science and technology is often blurred. This will quickly lead to the realization that technology permeates modern society, from little things that everyone takes for granted, such as pencil and paper, to major projects, such as dams and rocket launches.

A technologically literate person should be familiar with basic concepts important to technology. When engineers speak of a system, for instance, they mean components that work together to provide a desired function. Systems appear everywhere in technology, from a simple system, such as the half-dozen components in a click-and-write ballpoint pen, to complex systems with millions of components, assembled in hundreds of subsystems, such as commercial jetliners. Systems can also be scattered geographically, such as the roads, bridges, tunnels, signage, fueling stations, automobiles, and equipment that comprise, support, use, and help maintain our network of highways.

BOX 1-1 Characteristics of a Technologically Literate Citizen

Knowledge
- Recognizes the pervasiveness of technology in everyday life.
- Understands basic engineering concepts and terms, such as systems, constraints, and trade-offs.
- Is familiar with the nature and limitations of the engineering design process.
- Knows some of the ways technology shapes human history and people shape technology.
- Knows that all technologies entail risk, some that can be anticipated and some that cannot.
- Appreciates that the development and use of technology involve trade-offs and a balance of costs and benefits.
- Understands that technology reflects the values and culture of society.

Ways of Thinking and Acting
- Asks pertinent questions, of self and others, regarding the benefits and risks of technologies.
- Seeks information about new technologies.
- Participates, when appropriate, in decisions about the development and use of technology.

Capabilities
- Has a range of hands-on skills, such as using a computer for word processing and surfing the Internet and operating a variety of home and office appliances.
- Can identify and fix simple mechanical or technological problems at home or work.
- Can apply basic mathematical concepts related to probability, scale, and estimation to make informed judgments about technological risks and benefits.

Technologically literate people should also know something about the engineering design process. The goal of technological design is to meet certain criteria within various constraints, such as time deadlines, financial limits, or the need to avoid damaging the environment. Technologically literate people recognize that there is no such thing as a perfect design. All final designs inevitably involve trade-offs. Even if a design meets its stated criteria, there is no guarantee that the resulting technology will actually achieve the desired outcome because unexpected—often undesirable—consequences sometimes occur alongside intended ones. These include obvious things, such as the annoyance we all experience from mistakenly activated car alarms, to more serious things, such as repetitive-motion syndrome from heavy use of computer keyboards.

A technologically literate person recognizes that technology influences changes in society and has done so throughout history. In fact, many historical eras are identified by their dominant technology—Stone Age, Iron Age, Bronze Age, Industrial Age, Information Age. Technology-driven changes have been particularly evident in the past century. Automobiles have created a more mobile, spread-out society; aircraft and improved communications have led to a "smaller" world and, eventually, globalization; contraception has revolutionized sexual mores; and improved sanitation, agriculture, and medicine have extended life expectancy. A technologically literate person recognizes the role of technology in these changes and accepts the reality that the future will be different from the present largely because of technologies now coming into existence, from Internet-based activities to genetic engineering and cloning.

> There is nothing inevitable about the changes influenced by technology— they are the result of human decisions and not of impersonal historical forces.

The technologically literate person also recognizes that society shapes technology as much as technology shapes society. There is nothing inevitable about the changes influenced by technology—they are the result of human decisions and not of impersonal historical forces. The key people in successful technological innovation are not only engineers and scientists, but also designers and marketing specialists. New technologies must meet the requirements of consumers, business people, bankers, judges, environmentalists, politicians, and government bureaucrats (Bucciarelli, 1996). An electric car that no one buys might just as well never have been developed. A genetically engineered crop that is banned by the government is of little more use than the weeds in the fields. In short, many factors shape technology, and human beings, acting alone or in groups, determine the direction of technological development.

Technologically literate people realize that the use of any technology entails risk (Copp and Zanella, 1992; Gould et al., 1988). Some risks are obvious and well documented, such as the tens of thousands of deaths each year in the United States from automobile crashes. Others are more insidious and difficult to predict, such as the growth of algae in lakes and other bodies of water caused by the runoff of fertilizer from farms.

Technologically literate people will understand that *all* technologies, not just the obviously risky ones, have benefits and costs that must be weighed against one another. A new refining process may produce fewer waste products but may be more expensive than the old process. A new software program may have more features but may be more prone to failure than the old one and may also require learning a new system. Preservatives extend the shelf-life and improve the safety of our food but also cause allergic reactions in a small percentage of individuals.

Technologically literate people will recognize that sometimes there are risks to *not* using a technology. For example, consider the use of the pesticide DDT, a chemical technology for pest control. Because of DDT's effectiveness against mosquitoes, it is one of the most potent antimalaria weapons. In the 1970s, the use of DDT was banned in the United States and many other western nations, where there is no malaria to speak of, because of concerns about its effect on the environment. Farmers and others now use less environmentally questionable chemicals that were available at the time or that have been developed since to control insect pests.

But the withdrawal of DDT from malaria-endemic regions of the world has had serious consequences. In the East African island nation of Madagascar, for instance, the use of DDT was halted in 1986 after many years of successful control of malaria. By 1988, the incidence of the disease had increased dramatically, resulting in 100,000 deaths. When spraying with DDT was reinstituted, the incidence of malaria dropped by more than 90 percent in just 2 years (Roberts et al., 2000). The United Nations recently recognized the importance of DDT to public health in a treaty banning a number of persistent organic pollutants (UNEP, 2001).

The ability to use quantitative reasoning skills, especially skills related to probability, scale, and estimation, is critical to making informed judgments about technological risk. For example, based on the number of fatalities per mile traveled, a technologically literate person can make a reasonable judgment about whether it is riskier to travel from St. Louis to New York on a commercial airliner or by car.

Technologically literate people will appreciate that technologies are neither good nor evil, despite our tendency to invest them with these qualities. For example, the wide availability of handguns, as well as the desire of some to limit their availability, is an issue fraught with sociological, legal, public health, and economic considerations. Some people favor easy availability based on a need for self-defense, others favor limiting availability because of accidental deaths caused by handguns. In either case, weapons technology is not at fault.

Every technology reflects the values and culture of society. For instance, the popularity of cell phones in the United States is driven partly by the desire for the freedom to communicate at any time from virtually any location. Similar motivations, based on our historic emphasis on individuality and independence, have encouraged the use of private automobiles for transportation. The influence of values and culture on technology is often less straightforward. Technological development sometimes favors the values of certain groups more than others, for example the values of men more than those of women, which might explain why the initial designs of car air bags were not appropriate to the smaller stature of most women. (See "On or Off: Deciding About Your Car Air Bag," p. 26.)

> Every technology reflects the values and culture of society.

Once a person has a basic understanding of technology, he or she can educate himself or herself about particular technological issues. Technologically literate people will know how to extract the most important points from a newspaper story or a television interview or discussion, ask relevant questions, and make sense of the answers (Box 1-2).

A technologically literate individual should also have some hands-on capabilities with common, everyday technologies. At home and in the

---

BOX 1-2 Asking Questions About Technology

- What are the short-term and long-term risks of developing or using the technology?
- What are the costs of not developing or using the technology?
- Who will have access to the technology?
- Who will control it?
- Who will benefit and who will lose by the technology?
- What will the impact of the technology be on me, my family, and my community?

workplace, there are real benefits of knowing how to diagnose and even fix certain types of problems, such as resetting a tripped circuit breaker, replacing the battery in a smoke detector, or unjamming a food disposal unit. These tasks are not particularly difficult, but they require some basic knowledge and—in some cases—familiarity with simple hand tools. The same can be said for knowing how to remove and change a flat tire or hook up a new computer or phone. In addition, a level of comfort with personal computers and the software they use, and being able to surf the Internet, are essential to technological literacy.

Finally, a technologically literate person will be able to participate responsibly in debates or discussions about technological matters. When necessary, he or she will be able to take part in a public forum, communicate with city council members or members of Congress, and in other ways make his or her opinion heard on issues involving technology. Technological literacy does not specify a person's opinion. Literate citizens can and do hold quite different opinions depending upon the question at hand and their own values and judgment. A technologically literate individual will be able to envision how technology—in conjunction with, for example, the law or the marketplace—might help solve a problem.

Technical Competency

Technological literacy is not the same as technical competency. Technically trained people have a high level of knowledge and skill related to one or more specific technologies or technical areas. For instance, we expect people who repair appliances to be able to diagnose and fix mechanical or electrical problems in stoves, refrigerators, and dishwashers. A technician operating a computer numerically controlled milling machine must be knowledgeable about the technical aspects of the milling machine, as well as how the mill's operation fits into the larger manufacturing process. Civil engineers must have a detailed understanding of the behavior of structures and materials under load; mechanical engineers must have an in-depth understanding of mechanical systems and their applications; electrical engineers must be able to design and analyze electrical circuits. All of these jobs and many others require technically competent people— people with technical proficiency in a certain technological area, although not generally in other areas of technology.

A technologically literate person will not necessarily require ex-

> Technological literacy is not the same as technical competency.

BOX 1-3   What Would You Do?

Imagine yourself in California in the year 2003. A proposition on the statewide ballot calls for 10 percent of the cars sold in California to be powered by fuel cells or fuel-cell/internal combustion hybrids by the year 2007. Proponents claim this would reduce automobile-generated pollution and force the rapid development of a more environmentally friendly technology, which, given this initial boost, can then take over a larger and larger market share on its own. Opponents respond that the automobile industry cannot produce safe fuel-cell-powered cars by 2007, that the cars will have to be subsidized or no one will buy them, and that, anyway, most of the vehicle-generated pollution comes from tractor-trailers, not modern cars, which already have a lot of pollution-control equipment. How do you go about deciding which way to vote?

tensive technical skills. Technological literacy is more a capacity to understand the broader technological world rather than an ability to work with specific pieces of it. Some familiarity with at least a few technologies will be useful, however, as a concrete basis for thinking about technology. Someone who is knowledgeable about the history of technology and about basic technological principles but who has no hands-on capabilities with even the most common technologies cannot be as technologically literate as someone who has those capabilities.

But specialized technical skills do not guarantee technological literacy. Workers who know every operational detail of an air conditioner or who can troubleshoot a software glitch in a personal computer may not have a sense of the risks, benefits, and trade-offs associated with technological developments generally and may be poorly prepared to make choices about other technologies that affect their lives. For example, they might not be well prepared to decide if a car powered by a gas-electric hybrid engine is a good investment, and if it would be better for the environment than a traditionally powered car (Box 1-3).

Even engineers, who have traditionally been considered experts in technology, may not have the training or experience necessary to think about the social, political, and ethical implications of their work and so may not be technologically literate. The broad perspective on technology implied by technological literacy would be as valuable to engineers and other technical specialists as to people with no direct involvement in the development or production of technology.

Conclusion

A full appreciation of technological literacy, as of technology itself, requires an understanding of the larger society and culture in which it exists. Like other types of literacy, technological literacy is intimately related to many aspects of our lives. The capability dimension of technological literacy, for instance, requires a hands-on, design, and problem-solving orientation, which is in keeping with the job requirements for many workers, in both technical and nontechnical fields. The knowledge dimension of technological literacy is related to other academic areas, such as science, mathematics, history, and language arts. In fact, technological literacy could be a thematic unifier for many subjects now taught separately in American schools. The thinking and action dimension of technological literacy places it squarely in the realm of democracy and civics. Some level of participation in decision making about the development and use of technology is an essential aspect of technological literacy.

References

AAAS (American Association for the Advancement of Science). 1990a. The Nature of Technology and The Designed World. Chapters 3 and 8 in Science for All Americans. Washington, D.C.: AAAS.

AAAS. 1990b. Habits of Mind. Chapter 12 in Science for All Americans. Washington, D.C.: AAAS.

AAAS. 1993. Benchmarks for Science Literacy. New York: Oxford University Press.

Bucciarelli, L. 1996. Designing Engineers. Cambridge, Mass.: MIT Press.

Copp, N.H., and A. Zanella. 1992. Discovery, Innovation, and Risk: Case Studies in Science and Technology (New Liberal Arts). Cambridge, Mass.: MIT Press.

CPEMST (Commission on Precollege Education in Mathematics, Science and Technology). 1983. Educating Americans for the 21st Century: A Plan of Action for Improving Mathematics, Science and Technology Education for All American Elementary and Secondary Students So That Their Achievement Is the Best in the World by 1995: A Report to the American People and the National Science Board. Washington, D.C.: National Science Board Commission on Precollege Education in Mathematics, Science and Technology.

DoEd (U.S. Department of Education). 1996. Getting America's Students Ready for the 21st Century: Meeting the Technology Literacy Challenge. A Report to the Nation on Technology and Education. Washington, D.C.: DoEd.

Dyrenfurth, M.J. 1991. Technological literacy synthesized. Pp. 138–183 in Technological Literacy. Council on Technology Teacher Education, 40th Yearbook, edited by M.J. Dyrenfurth and M.R. Kozak. Peoria, Ill.: Macmillan/McGraw-Hill, Glencoe Division.

Fanning, J. 2001. Expanding the Definition of Technological Literacy in Schools. Available online at: <http://www.mcrel.org/products/noteworthy/noteworthy/jimf.asp> (November 13, 2001).

Gould, L.C., G.T. Gardner, D.R. DeLuca, A.R. Tiemann, L.W. Doob, and J.A.J. Stolwijk. 1988. Perceptions of Technological Risks and Benefits. New York: Russell Sage.

Hirsch, E.D., Jr. 1988. Cultural Literacy: What Every American Needs to Know. New York: Vintage Books.

ITEA (International Technology Education Association). 2000. Preparing students for a technological world. Pp. 1–10 in Standards for Technological Literacy: Content for the Study of Technology. Reston, Virginia.: ITEA.

Madison, J. 1822. Letter to W.T. Barry, August 4, 1822. P. 276 in The Writings of James Madison, Vol. 3, edited by G. Hunt. New York: G.P. Putnam's Sons.

Mitchem, C. 1994. Thinking Through Technology: The Path Between Engineering and Philosophy. Chicago: University of Chicago Press.

Roberts, D.R., S. Manguin, and J. Mouchet. 2000. DDT house spraying and re-emerging malaria. Lancet 356:330–332.

21st Century Workforce Commission. 2000. A Nation of Opportunity—Building America's 21st Century Workforce. Washington, D.C.: U.S. Department of Labor.

UNEP (United Nations Environment Programme). 2001. Text of Persistent Organic Pollutants Treaty Concluded in Johannesburg; Signing Conference Set for Stockholm 22 to 23 May 2001. Press release. Available online at: <http://www.chem.unep.ch/pops/POPs_Inc/press_releases/pressrel-01/pr5-01.htm> (November 12, 2001).

2
Benefits of
Technological Literacy

The argument for technological literacy is rooted in a single, fundamental belief. In a world permeated by technology, an individual can function more effectively if he or she is familiar with and has a basic understanding of technology. A higher level of technological literacy in the United States would have a number of benefits, for individuals and for the society as a whole.

Improving Decision Making

Technological literacy prepares individuals to make well-informed choices in their role as consumers. The world is full of products and services that promise to make people's lives easier, more enjoyable, more efficient, or healthier, and more and more of these products appear every year. A technologically literate person cannot know how each new technology works, its advantages and disadvantages, how to operate it, and so on, but he or she can learn enough about a product to put it to good use or to choose not to use it.

Americans are not only consumers; they are also workers, members of families and communities, and citizens of a large, complex democracy. In all of these spheres, they face personal decisions that involve the development or use of technology. Is a local referendum on issuing bonds for the construction of a new power plant a wise use of taxpayer dollars? Does a plan to locate a new waste incinerator within several miles of one's home pose serious health risks, as opponents of the initiative may claim? How should one react to efforts by local government to place surveillance cameras in high-crime areas of the city? Technologically literate people will be much better able to address these and many other technology-related questions.

Decision making is not only personal. Leaders in a variety of sectors, including business, government, and the media, make decisions daily that affect what others—sometimes thousands or even millions of people—think and do. These individuals in particular will benefit from a considerable understanding of the nature of technology, and an awareness that all technologies involve trade-offs and may result in unintended consequences. With a higher level of technological literacy in the nation, people in positions of power will be more likely to manage technological developments in a way that maximizes the benefits to humankind and minimizes the negative impacts. Of course, there is no hard-and-fast line between purely personal concerns and business interests, the needs of states, and the needs of the nation. In most cases the personal interests of everyday Americans do influence decisions by policy makers and company CEOs.

Some concrete examples can illustrate the importance of techno-logical literacy to decision making at all levels. The next three sections present descriptions of current issues that require decision making of some sort. The first is the use of car air bags and relates mostly to the concerns of individual citizens. The second addresses genetically modified foods, an issue relevant to individuals, who must decide which foods to buy at the grocery store; policy makers, who must take into account regulatory, trade, and other considerations; and the biotechnology industry and farmers, the two groups most responsible for creating and selling such products. The third example is the California energy crisis, which has put pressure on individuals, businesses, and political leaders to develop short-term and long-term solutions.

All three examples have a central technological component, which may be part of the problem, part of a solution, or both. The technological component cannot be separated from political, legal, social, and other concerns. A box at the end of each example shows how the three dimensions of technological literacy—knowledge, capabilities, and ways of thinking and acting—might come into play in each case.

On or Off? Deciding About Your Car Air Bag

By now, almost everyone knows that car air bags can cause injury or even death, as well as offer protection. Most car owners are aware of

> There is no hard-and-fast line between purely personal concerns and business interests, the needs of states, and the needs of the nation.

recommendations by safety experts that young children be placed in the back seat and that a distance of at least 10 inches be maintained between the driver and the steering wheel to minimize the chances of air bag-induced injury. Some people feel that air bags are not worth the risk and would like to shut them off, or at least have the option to do so. An on-off switch can be installed, but it requires permission from the National Highway Traffic Safety Administration (NHTSA) and costs several hundred dollars.

The decision to disable your air bag has potentially serious consequences. To make the best choice, the decision maker should know something about how air bags work, how well they protect, and in what situations.

All air bag systems operate in basically the same way. Onboard sensing devices measure crash impact. Once activated, the crash sensors signal solid-propellant inflators to begin the chemical reaction that generates nitrogen gas that fills the air bag. The gas inflates a folded nylon bag, which acts as a protective cushion between the occupant and the inside of the car. As the person collides with the air bag, vents in the bag allow the gas to escape, absorbing energy and reducing the severity of impact. Ideally, occupants collide with the bag just as it becomes fully inflated. But if the bag strikes the occupant while it is still inflating, it can cause serious injury or death because the bags travel at speeds of more than 100 mph.

Studies show that air bags are about 13 percent effective in saving the lives of drivers not wearing a lap-shoulder seat belt (NHTSA, 1996). That is, if 100 fatally injured drivers in cars without air bags had been driving cars with air bags, 13 of them would have survived. By comparison, seat belts are approximately 42 percent effective in preventing driver fatalities, compared to situations in which no seat belts are worn. The combined effectiveness, for drivers, of seat belts and air bags is 47 percent. This means that, overall, air bags reduce the risk of death for drivers wearing seat belts by 9 percent ([58 − 53]/58).

Overall, air bags reduce the risk of death for drivers wearing seat belts by 9 percent.

As it turns out, the government vastly overestimated the effectiveness of air bags, claiming in the late 1970s they would save 12,000 lives *annually* (Federal Register, 1977). The actual record is not nearly as impressive. From 1986 through April 2001, fewer than 7,000 lives had been saved by air bags. An estimated 246 people (including 61 unconfirmed air bag-related fatalities), mostly drivers and children, had been killed by air bags during the same period (GAO, 2001a). By comparison, about 11,000 lives are saved every year by seat belts.

The benefits of air bags depend on many factors. One of the most important factors is the weight and, especially, the height of the occupants. Because those two parameters are closely linked to gender, the effectiveness of air bags differs greatly for men and women. For example, nearly three-quarters of the drivers killed by air bags were women. In one study, air bags used in conjunction with seat belts reduced total harm (a mix of fatalities and injuries) among male drivers by 11 percent but increased the harm to female drivers wearing seat belts by 9 percent (Dalmotas et al., 1996). For people of small stature (shorter than 5 feet, 3 inches tall), air bags increased total harm. The data also show that age makes a difference. Drivers between the ages of 15 and 50 wearing seat belts were better protected with air bags. However, no clear evidence showed added protection for belted drivers over the age of 50.

A number of factors besides air bags affect the safety of vehicle occupants. Consider the 9 percent figure, which represents the additional lifesaving potential of air bags for belted drivers. A belted driver could reduce his or her risk of dying in a crash by the same amount by driving a car 200 pounds heavier (Evans, 1991). The same nine-percent reduction in driver fatalities could be achieved across the nation by lowering average driving speeds on U.S. roads by 2 mph.

Recently, the technological landscape for air bags has begun to change. New NHTSA regulations require that automakers design and install more advanced air bag systems for model 2004 vehicles. The new devices are meant to meet the safety needs of drivers and passengers of different sizes, weights, and seating positions. The rules have stimulated millions of dollars of research on occupant classification sensors, seat belt usage sensors, multistage inflators that can fill air bags at varying rates, and less aggressive air bag designs (GAO, 2001a).

Return now to the original decision—whether or not to install an on-off switch. The decision will depend on many factors related not only to the personal characteristics of the people who will use the vehicle—drivers and passengers—but also to the type and age of the vehicle itself. To make an intelligent choice, the individual will have to draw on all three dimensions of technological literacy (Box 2-1).

A number of factors besides air bags affect the safety of vehicle occupants.

BOX 2-1   The Technologically Literate Citizen and Air Bags

Knowledge
- Understands that for many occupants air bags provide a moderate increase in safety over the use of seat belts alone.
- Appreciates that there are risks to turning off the air-bag switch, just as there are risks associated with leaving the air-bag system intact.
- Understands that more advanced air-bag systems will probably be more expensive than the old ones, adding to the overall cost of the car.
- Understands that, as certain technologies like air bags become more sophisticated, the incidence of mechanical, electrical, or other problems may increase.
- Understands that there may be unforeseen consequences with the new air-bag systems, some of which may require modifications of the existing technology or entirely new technological solutions.

Ways of Thinking and Acting
- Takes steps (e.g., online or library research and reading; contacting state or federal auto safety or consumer organizations) to learn about the pros and cons of air bags.
- Itemizes personal and vehicle-specific factors to determine the appropriateness of an on-off switch for his or her car.
- When buying a new car with an advanced air-bag system, inquires about the risks of the system, especially related to the age and size of front-seat occupants.

Capabilities
- Can optimize the safety and effectiveness of air bags, for example by seating children in the back seat and maintaining an appropriate distance between the steering wheel and driver.
- Can apply for permission to have the switch installed and to identify and interact with a qualified mechanic to have the work done.
- Is comfortable knowing when and how to turn the switch on and off.

Waiter, There's a GMO in My Soup

In fall 2000, American consumers were informed that a type of genetically modified corn approved for use in animal feed had somehow made its way into grocery stores as an ingredient in taco shells manufactured by Kraft Foods. There were concerns that a bacterial protein inserted into the corn's genetic makeup to protect growing plants from the European corn borer could trigger an allergic reaction in some people. Kraft recalled millions of its taco shells in response (*Washington Post*, September 18, 2000).

Groups opposed to genetically modified foods cited the episode as evidence that the risks had not been taken seriously enough. The biotechnology industry downplayed the importance of the mix-up, pointing out that the same protein is present in other types of corn grown for human consumption—including organically grown corn—and noting that the amount of modified corn was so small that it was unlikely to cause any noticeable health effects. The media and the public were left to flounder in a sea of conflicting opinions and interpretations.

In early 2001, batches of seed corn grown by U.S. farmers and slated for sale overseas were found to contain small amounts of the same genetically modified version discovered in taco shells (*Washington Post*, March 1, 2001). Because European and Asian opposition to genetically modified organisms (GMOs) is very strong (Laget and Cantley, 2001), billions of dollars of U.S. exports were threatened. The U.S. government ended up buying back millions of dollars worth of seed stock that had been mixed with the genetically modified version, called StarLink.

> Because European and Asian opposition to genetically modified organisms is very strong, billions of dollars of U.S. exports were threatened.

In late July 2001, a scientific advisory panel to the Environmental Protection Agency (EPA) concluded there was not enough evidence to prove that the modified corn does not pose an allergic risk to people. Based on the panel's finding, the agency decided to maintain its policy of banning even trace amounts of the modified corn in foods (*Washington Post*, July 28, 2001).

Because of fears of adverse health effects, the European Union (EU) had already effectively banned the importation of most biotech-derived foods in 1998, causing sales of exported U.S. corn to plunge from about $300 million annually in the mid-1990s to less than $10 million in recent years (GAO, 2001b). The EU accounts for only about 5 percent of the market for this U.S. crop, but other larger markets in Asia and Latin America have also taken steps, such as requiring labeling of genetically modified food products, that are expected to decrease the size of the export market for American farmers.

Perhaps no technology better illustrates the current mismatch between the adoption of a new technology and society's ability to deal with it. In the past 10 years, the idea of taking genes from one organism and transferring them into another has gone from a laboratory demonstration to a commercial reality. In 1999, U.S. farmers planted some 70 million acres of genetically engineered crops, including 36 percent of all corn, 55 percent of soybeans, and 43 percent of cotton. Most of those crops were modified either to produce a substance, often a protein, that defends them against insect pests—as was the case for the corn that ended up in the tacos—or else to be resistant to herbicides that are sprayed on the fields to control weeds (*New York Times*, March 14, 2000).

In the next decade, we could see explosive growth in the agricultural uses of genetic engineering. Researchers are constantly improving techniques for putting new genes into organisms, and scientists can now map out entire genomes—that is, the entire genetic makeup of organisms—quickly and at relatively low cost. This will have two effects. First, it will improve our understanding of the genetics of crops and farm animals. Second, it will provide a multitude of new genes to work with.

In the United States, the genetically engineered changes benefit both farmers and the environment. In the case of StarLink, for example, farmers growing the modified corn can use less chemical pesticide, thus cutting their production costs and, at the same time, reducing harmful pesticide-laden runoff. In developing countries, however, the benefits could be even greater. Genetic enhancements could mean the difference between starvation and survival for large numbers of people and between dependency on foreign imports and agricultural self-sufficiency for entire nations.

Some gene splicing dramatically improves the health benefits of foods. In Switzerland, for instance, a German scientist, Ingo Potrykus, has engineered a new type of rice that produces generous amounts of beta carotene, which the human body turns into Vitamin A. If widely adopted, this so-called golden rice could prevent 1 to 2 million deaths and 500,000 cases of blindness each year among children who survive almost completely on rice for months at a time and suffer from Vitamin A deficiency. Healthier foods of this sort could enhance diets and improve health around the world, in both developed and developing countries.

It is impossible to know whether a technologically literate population would reject GMOs, embrace them, or find a middle ground.

Today, we find ourselves with a volatile combination of rapidly growing biotech capabilities and a public that is not prepared to understand or assess those capabilities. In Europe, the mismatch has led to a nearly complete ban on genetically modified foodstuffs. Ingo Potrykus's plan to distribute his beta-carotene rice to poor farmers around the world is threatened by an effort in Switzerland to pass legislation forbidding the export of GMOs.

The development and use of GMOs raises a number of questions, not only for consumers but also for farmers and policy makers. Which foods are safe to eat? Which crops should be grown and under what conditions and to whom can they be sold? How should products containing GMOs be labeled? It is impossible to know whether a technologically literate population would reject GMOs, embrace them, or find a middle ground, accepting foods that provided significant improvements, such as the beta-carotene rice, but rejecting foods that simply lowered the cost of production by a few percentage points. Whatever the outcome, the

---

BOX 2-2 The Technologically Literate Citizen and GMOs

Knowledge

- Understands that a common method of creating genetically modified organisms (GMOs) involves transferring genetic material from one organism to another.
- Knows that genetic engineering has been used for decades to produce or enhance food crops, chemicals, drugs and other therapeutics, and organisms with special characteristics, such as oil-eating bacteria.
- Recognizes that health and environmental risks might be associated with some GMOs and that some of the risks are uncertain or unknown.
- Understands that one trade-off of producing GMOs may be a decrease in export opportunities for U.S. crops and food products.
- Appreciates that the development and use of GMOs has economic and political effects in the United States as well as internationally.

Ways of Thinking and Acting

- Monitors and, when appropriate, participates in decisions by federal and state agencies, as well as by local grocery stores, regarding the sale of GMO-containing foods.
- Uses information on product labels and in advertising to make informed decisions about purchasing and consuming GMO-containing foods.

Capabilities

- Can critically evaluate news coverage regarding the scale and probability of risks associated with GMOs.

decision should be made by people with a basic understanding of technology and an ability to weigh risks and benefits (Box 2-2).

Turning the Lights Out: The California Energy Crisis

In January 2001, California was facing an energy crisis. Demand for electric power had grown to the point that the state's two major utilities, Pacific Gas & Electric and Southern California Edison, were having difficulty meeting the need. On days of particularly high demand, they instituted rolling blackouts, turning off electricity to first one area, then another. In addition, the utilities were losing money so rapidly that both were predicting bankruptcy.

How did California, which would have the world's sixth largest economy if it were a country, get into this predicament? The answer is complex. At least a part of the explanation is the failure of state officials to understand—or perhaps their decision to ignore—basic facts about how the electric power industry works. The state also appears to have miscalculated when it deregulated the electric power industry. In addition, uncontrollable factors, such as the pace of economic growth in California, and drought and colder than average temperatures in the Northwest, conspired to put further pressure on the system.

Commercial electricity is generated in plants large enough to provide energy for tens of thousands of homes. All electricity, whether generated from hydroelectric dams, solar collectors, wind turbines, or plants that consume coal, oil, natural gas, or nuclear fuel, is fed into a network of transmission wires—the "grid"—which delivers the power where it is needed. Operators keep track of demand on an hourly basis, making sure that enough power is being fed into the system. If demand outstrips supply, the operators attempt to find extra power from outside plants attached to the grid. If they cannot, they shut off power to some customers to prevent the entire system from failing.

Once it enters the grid, there is no distinction between electricity generated by, say, a natural gas plant outside Sacramento and a nuclear plant near San Diego. In short, electricity becomes a commodity that can be bought and sold by the kilowatt-hour. Because of this, a company like Southern California Edison does not have to generate exactly enough power for its customers. If it needs more, the company can buy extra power from another producer; if it has extra power, it can sell it.

For decades the electric power industry has been closely regulated by the states. Each utility was required to have enough generating capacity to serve its customers. In turn, the state set rates for electricity that guaranteed the utilities a reasonable return on their investment. Although this was a safe arrangement for the utilities, some critics argued that regulation removed much of the utilities' incentive to produce power at the lowest possible cost.

In response to these arguments, the state of California decided in 1996 to deregulate its electric utilities. According to the plan devised by legislators, the two major utilities would sell off much of their generating capacity and buy electric power wholesale from whatever companies would provide it to them at the lowest cost (*New York Times*, January 2, 2001). The idea was that competition would drive prices down, and the utilities would be able to purchase power at a lower cost than the cost of producing it. At a second, later stage, the retail market would be deregulated, allowing consumers to benefit from the lower costs of electricity production.

As events would prove, the plan had at least two major flaws.

> Once it enters the grid, there is no distinction between electricity generated by a natural gas plant outside Sacramento and a nuclear plant near San Diego.

First, it did not pay enough attention to the building of new generating plants. In the early 1990s, California had an excess of electrical generating capacity, and its economy was growing slowly enough that new plants did not seem to be a priority (*New York Times*, January 11, 2001). Pacific Gas & Electric and Southern California Edison had always provided enough electricity, and the lawmakers who wrote the bill assumed that, with deregulation, other companies would build whatever plants were necessary (*New York Times*, January 5, 2001).

But they had not counted on the hurdles these companies would face. California's environmental laws are among the nation's toughest, so building new plants is more difficult there than in many other states (*New York Times*, January 10, 11, 2001). Those difficulties, combined with uncertainties about how the deregulated industry would work, made companies cautious about committing to new plants. And those that did commit found that the approval rate was slowed both by the state agencies that approve new plants and local activist groups that did not want generating plants built in their backyards (*New York Times*, January 5, 11, 12, 2001). As a result, in the 3 years after the deregulation law passed, California added only 2 percent to its generating capacity (*New York Times*, January 11, 2001).

> In the 3 years after the deregulation law passed, California added only 2 percent to its generating capacity.

Meanwhile, the California economy grew rapidly, twice the national average in the late 1990s, and demand for electricity grew apace (*New York Times*, January 11, 2001). By summer 2000, demand had caught up with supply, and on hot days during peak hours, the demand exceeded maximum generating capacity. The utilities were forced to buy electricity from outside the state, but other Western states had little to spare, and the scarcity drove prices up sharply. The California utilities, which had been accustomed to paying about $60 to $70 per megawatt-hour, suddenly found themselves paying as much as $750, the federally mandated maximum. Later, when the cap was removed, they were forced to pay spot prices as high as $1,400 per megawatt-hour.

This increased cost could not be passed on to consumers, however, which was a second major flaw in the deregulation plan. According to the 1996 law, retail prices of electricity were not scheduled to be deregulated until March 2002; until then, the utilities could charge no more than $65 per megawatt-hour (*New York Times*, January 4, 2001). As a result, Pacific Gas & Electric and Southern California Edison found themselves paying out several times as much to buy power as they took in for selling it; by January 2001, they had lost a combined $12 billion.

Unable to pay their bills and unable to find creditors willing to lend them the billions they needed to keep going, both utilities warned they might go bankrupt by February.

The price freeze also meant that consumers, who were paying an artificially low price for energy, had no incentive to use less electricity. As a result, demand continued to rise. The only exception was in the San Diego area, where San Diego Gas & Electric had sold all of its power plants and was free to raise its retail rates in response to wholesale costs. In the summer of 2000, when that utility more than doubled its rates, consumer energy use dropped by more than 5 percent in a few weeks (*New York Times*, January 10, 2001).

The California energy crisis illustrates the danger of taking a technology for granted and acting without thinking carefully about the factors that influence the technology in question. A more technologically literate California legislator might have insisted that planning for additional generating capacity begin before deregulation went forward. The trade-offs between increasing electricity supply and protecting the environment may also have been more prominent in the state's debate on energy policy. More knowledgeable citizens might have made a difference, too, for instance by being more supportive of proposals for building new generating plants, agreeing to stricter conservation measures, or pushing for more investment in alternative energy sources, such as solar, wind, and thermal power. If lawmakers had believed their constituents were technologically savvy enough to understand the need for steps like these, they might have been more confident about making politically unpopular, but necessary, decisions.

> A more technologically literate California legislator might have insisted that planning for additional generating capacity begin before deregulation went forward.

Even after the crisis had begun, a more technologically literate public might have made a difference. Much of the debate over the crisis ignored the fact that the utilities had enough power except during times of peak load—the hours when demand is at or near a maximum. If consumers had been convinced to cut their usage slightly during those hours, the utilities might not have been forced to buy electricity at inflated prices.

Based on the three dimensions of technological literacy, we can suggest the kinds of understanding and competencies technologically literate Californians—legislators and citizens—might have brought to bear on the state's energy crisis (Box 2-3). It is impossible to know, of course, whether the crisis could have been avoided if the level of technological literacy had been higher. It seems reasonable, however, that the

> **BOX 2-3   The Technologically Literate Citizen and California's Energy Crisis**
>
> **Knowledge**
> - Understands electricity can be generated in a number of ways, each of which has advantages and disadvantages.
> - Understands that electricity is transported from one place to another as a commodity and is sold through an interstate grid.
> - Understands that many factors besides technology, such as politics, regulations, and markets, determine energy supply and demand.
> - Understands that it takes many years to create new generating capacity.
>
> **Ways of Thinking and Acting**
> - Takes advantage of opportunities for conserving electricity at home and work.
> - Keeps abreast of the short-term and long-term proposals for ensuring stable supplies of electricity.
> - Evaluates these proposals in terms of their potential risks, benefits, costs, and the constraints to their development.
>
> **Capabilities**
> - Can evaluate the costs and benefits of energy-efficient appliances and fuel-efficient vehicles.
> - Can change a light bulb, set the thermostat on a furnace or air conditioning unit to conserve energy, and locate and fix a tripped circuit breaker in the event of a power outage.

debate over electric power in California would have been different and might have included more prominently the voices of everyday citizens.

Increasing Citizen Participation

In addition to being consumers and workers, Americans are also citizens of a democracy who have a right—indeed a responsibility—to let their voices be heard on matters that concern them. Most current political, legal, and ethical issues, from what to do about global warming to how to protect privacy in the Information Age, have a technological component. A technologically literate citizen is likely to participate in the decision making, whether by voting for a candidate or in a referendum, writing a letter to the editor of a local paper, sending an e-mail to a member of Congress, participating in a public opinion poll, speaking out at a town meeting, or supporting the work of an organized special-interest group.

In a democratic society, people must be involved in the technological decisions that affect them for two very different reasons—one practical and one philosophical. First, decisions made without public input are often eventually rejected as illegitimate and antidemocratic, which can impede the acceptance of a technology. Second, democratic principles are based on citizen participation—at least indirect participation through elected representatives—in decisions that affect them. Few decisions today affect people more than those about the kinds of technologies that are developed and how they are used. Citizen input can be influential during the design or research and development (R&D) phase of technology. People can also affect how a technology is used once it passes into the public arena.

Public participation in discussions about the development and uses of technology is also important for another reason—it can lead to greater technological literacy. The simple act of asking and trying to answer questions about technology can lead to a better understanding not only of technical, but also of the social, economic, and political aspects of the issue at hand. What are the risks and benefits, and the trade-offs, of developing or using a technology? Who wins and who loses? What are the costs and the alternatives? Public involvement also gives policy makers a sense of their constituents' fears and hopes, and thus an indication of the public response to a particular path of technology development, as well as to new or lesser known alternatives.

> Few decisions today affect people more than those about the kinds of technologies that are developed and how they are used.

Slaying the "Green Snake" [1]

The design and construction of the Boston Central Artery and Tunnel, the largest public works project under way in the United States, illustrates the power of everyday people to influence the shape and direction of technological development.

Scheduled for completion in 2004, the $12 billion-plus project, involving 160 lane miles in a 7.5-mile corridor, will bring to a close the development of a massive interstate highway network begun during the administration of President Dwight Eisenhower. The central artery portion of the project will remove the "Green Snake," the elevated roadway that has been an enormous eyesore in the heart of downtown Boston. The Green Snake, which was built in 1959, is now clogged with almost three times as much traffic as planners originally anticipated. The Boston Central Artery and Tunnel will replace the elevated structure with an underground route that is expected to facilitate the movement of inter-

---

[1]This account of the Boston Central Artery and Tunnel is based on Hughes (1998).

state highway traffic through the Boston region. The harbor tunnel portion of the project will provide a route to Logan Airport. The project also calls for a new bridge across the Charles River from Boston into Cambridge.

The project is unique in the extent and nature of public participation during the design phase and the sensitivity to environmental concerns shown by the developers. Many people believe the project could become a model for other cities throughout the world.

Critics, however, point out that the actual cost of the project has greatly exceeded the original projected figure. Unanticipated construction problems can account for much of the cost overrun, but also to blame are the enormous expenses incurred in responding to the concerns of interest groups about potential environmental, economic, and cultural impacts on Boston.

Because the federal government funds about 90 percent of the work, the project had to comply with the National Environmental Protection Act of 1969, which requires the preparation of an Environmental Impact Statement (EIS). EISs are lengthy documents that identify in detail how a project will positively and negatively affect the environment. The EIS prepared for the Central Artery and Tunnel addressed 17 categories, including transportation, air quality, noise and vibration, energy, economic characteristics, visual characteristics, historic resources, water quality, wetlands and waterways, and vegetation and wildlife.

Because the law mandated public participation in the design of the project, a draft EIS was widely circulated by managers of the project. Copies were placed in libraries; a public hearing was held; and a public comment period was provided. One hundred seventy-five people, including spokespersons for government agencies, such as EPA, and public interest groups, including the Sierra Club, testified at the hearing, and 99 individuals provided written comments.

Even before the EIS was circulated, negotiations between project management and the public, especially neighborhood, business, and environmental groups, had resulted in a number of changes, called "mitigations," in the plan to address adverse impacts. Affluent organizations even hired their own engineers to provide detailed alternative designs for highway alignment, ramps, and locations of ventilation buildings. The citizens of East Boston called upon their congressional representatives to block funding for the project, if the harbor tunnel emerged in their neighborhood. The tunnel now emerges on Logan Airport property. Overall, the

The project is unique in the extent and nature of public participation during the design phase and the sensitivity to environmental concerns shown by the developers.

project has accommodated some 1,100 mitigations, which added an estimated $2.8 billion to the total cost.

In 1990, public attention was focused on the design for the Charles River bridge and ramps. The twenty-sixth alternative design, nicknamed Scheme Z, was announced in August 1988 but aroused little reaction, probably because three-dimensional models and easily comprehensible drawings of the design were not available. When a model of the structure was displayed a year later, the architectural critic of the *Boston Globe* compared the bridge and access ramps to a massive wall across the Charles River. An EPA official predicted that the structure would be the ugliest in New England.

Various citizen groups responded vociferously to Scheme Z. A newly formed organization, Citizens for a Livable Charlestown, joined the chorus of complaints and hired an artist to prepare an illustration emphasizing the overwhelming size of the bridge and associated roadways. Publication of the drawing in the *Charlestown Patriot* caused a public uproar. Within weeks, other groups, including the Charles River Watershed Association, which has more than 1,000 members, and the New England chapter of the Sierra Club joined the chorus of opposition. A weeklong series of articles in the *Boston Globe* in December 1990 stressing the potential noise, shadows, and blight of the enormous structure fanned the fires of discontent, demonstrating the effectiveness of an alliance of media and activist groups in stimulating public participation. In light of the growing opposition, the Boston City Council, by unanimous vote, declared its opposition to Scheme Z.

In January 1991, the Massachusetts secretary of transportation attempted to assuage various interest groups by establishing a Bridge Design Review Committee. The composition of the 42-member committee was based on current thinking about participatory design and conflict resolution. The committee's deliberations were open, multidisciplinary, and consensus seeking. Members represented national environmental organizations, such as the Sierra Club; local environmental, transportation, and business groups, such as the Charles River Watershed Association and the Boston Chamber of Commerce; and organizations of professional engineers, architects, and urban planners.

Instead of revising Scheme Z, in June 1991 the committee voted unanimously to abandon it and proposed a new conceptual design for a tunnel under the Charles River to replace some of the massive bridge structure. The Federal Highway Administration and the U.S. Army

> Overall, the project has accommodated some 1,100 mitigations, which added an estimated $2.8 billion to the total cost.

Corps of Engineers, however, called for other, nontunnel alternatives. Critics warned that digging for a tunnel would not only be expensive, but would also cause serious pollution problems for the river.

The conflict was resolved when the state selected a bridge designed by world-famous Swiss architect Christian Menn. The new design specified that two bridges be built side by side, one with 10 lanes, and one with 4. Peter Zuk, the Central Artery/Tunnel project director, proclaimed it a world-class, elegant design. Others characterized it as a signature structure, and an appropriate gateway to a great city.

The Boston project illustrates some interesting ideas about technological literacy. In this case it was primarily organizations, especially environmental organizations, not individuals, that were active, effective participants in design reviews, controversies, and the obtaining of mitigations. The public at large did not have to be knowledgeable about the technical details of highway construction and environmental impact. However, public support—financial and political—for the involved organizations was critical. In addition, the media, especially local newspapers, played a major role in informing the public and raising the level of concern.

Supporting a Modern Workforce

One of the obvious benefits of technological literacy is in the economic realm. Technology, particularly in the high-tech sector, has been driving much of the economic growth in the United States and elsewhere, and an increasing percentage of jobs require technological skills (Rausch, 1998). Although technological literacy and technical competency are not the same thing, they are related. Increasing the overall level of technological literacy would almost certainly improve the climate for technology-driven economic growth. A technologically literate population would, for example, understand that science and technology are the foundation of our economic strength and would be more likely to support the research, education, and economic policies that support that foundation. Conversely, technologically literate citizens would be less likely to support policies that would undermine the technological basis of the economy.

Improving technological literacy would also help to prepare individuals for jobs in our technology-driven economy, thus strengthening the economy. Technologically literate workers are more likely than those

Increasing the overall level of technological literacy would almost certainly improve the climate for technology-driven economic growth.

lacking such literacy to have a broad range of knowledge and abilities, such as the critical skills identified by the Secretary's Commission on Achieving Necessary Skills (SCANS) (DOL, 1991).

The study of technology involves evaluating how others have successfully solved problems and provides experience in hands-on problem solving; hence, technologically literate workers are likely to be able to identify and solve problems. They are also more likely to put things in a broad context, because the study of technology emphasizes systems thinking. They are more likely to be comfortable with complex interrelationships, which are common in technological systems. And they may be able to troubleshoot problems with equipment when necessary because they have learned how to ask the necessary questions to understand why a technology works—or why it isn't working.

Technology is everywhere in the business world. Doctors, nurses, and other medical personnel depend on a growing number of medical devices for examination, diagnosis, and treatment. Teachers are bombarded with new tools for preparing and delivering lessons, researching new teaching techniques, and enabling students to learn outside the traditional setting. Farmers use the Global Positioning System to help monitor crop yields and tailor the application of herbicides, and they must decide whether or not to plant genetically modified seeds. Self-employed workers must set up home offices and purchase and operate their own office technology. Technologically literate people will tend to be more comfortable dealing with technologies that their jobs demand and will find it easier to master new technologies as they come along.

The military is also becoming increasingly dependent on technology. The nation's 1.4 million soldiers, airmen, sailors, and marines must be able to operate and manage technically complex weaponry, transportation systems, and communications systems (DOD, 2001). The effectiveness of U.S. fighting forces depends largely on how well they do their jobs. Their performance, in turn, depends not only on their knowledge of the specific systems but also on their problem-solving, critical-thinking, and teamwork skills. Improving the overall technological literacy of the population will make it easier for the military to find men and women who can serve effectively.

Employers in all sectors are demanding workers with a mix of factual and conceptual knowledge, critical thinking skills, and procedural knowledge. In this climate, technologically literate workers may have a competitive advantage in the job market and may be more likely to land better paying, more interesting jobs. For similar reasons, technological literacy can help narrow the growing wage gap—and related shortage of skills—between salaried workers with higher educations and hourly workers without it (DOL, 1999).

At the moment, the United States does not produce enough technically skilled workers to support certain sectors of its high-tech economy. Therefore, we must depend on workers brought in from other countries (Committee on Workforce Needs in Information Technology, 2001; 21st Century Workforce Commission, 2000). A campaign for technological literacy could lessen our dependence on foreign workers by encouraging young students to pursue scientific or technical careers. Boosting the awareness of the importance of technology in the general population may increase the esteem and respect accorded to jobs in the technology sector, which would also encourage more students to pursue careers in science and engineering.

Narrowing the Digital Divide

Many commentators have noted a distressing pattern in the use of the Internet. Most of the people who have access to it, either at work or at home, and those most likely to know how to take advantage of its resources are more affluent, better educated, urban, and are not members of ethnic or racial minorities. The most recent data from the federal government show that this "digital divide" has been decreasing as Internet usage among most groups of Americans continues to increase (DOC, 2000). For instance, in rural areas, 39 percent of households had access to the Internet as of August 2000, a 75 percent jump from just 20 months earlier. The gap between the percentage of rural households with Internet access and the nationwide average fell from 4 percentage points to 2.6 percentage points in 2000, a drop of 35 percent.

Blacks and Hispanics have made significant gains in Internet access. Over the 20-month period, the proportion of black households with access increased from 11.2 percent to 23.5 percent; Hispanic access rose from 12.6 percent to 23.6 percent. However, large gaps still remain for these groups when measured against the national average, and these gaps appear to be growing. The gap in Internet access between black and Hispanic households and the national average was 18 percentage points in August 2000, an increase of 3 percentage points for blacks and 4.3 percentage points for Hispanics. Large gaps in the ownership of computers between these two groups and the national average of ownership have not narrowed since the last government survey.

Access to a personal computer is the single most important factor in whether or not a person uses the Internet. Not surprisingly, people in higher socioeconomic brackets are far more likely than those in lower brackets to have personal computers at home or have access to them at work. In addition, people with higher levels of education were more likely to use the Internet, regardless of their income level.

Black students are less likely than white students to own a home computer even when household incomes are factored into the equation. Furthermore, among those without home computers, black students are less likely than white students to access the Internet outside the home—in school, libraries, or friends' houses. As a result, many fewer black students than white students are working on the Internet.

A number of remedies have been suggested for closing the digital divide. Most focus on providing universal access to the Internet so that everyone can get online regardless of income level or job status. Equally important will be improving technological literacy because the better people understand the Internet and its value or are comfortable with technology, the more likely they will be to make the effort to learn to use it.

A similar situation exists for technology in general. All technology, not just computers and the Internet, empowers those who own it and understand it and puts those who do not at a disadvantage. Thus, the nation's poor and minorities will benefit much more by being technologically literate; being literate, they will find it easier to overcome their lack of preparation and participate effectively in an increasingly technological world.

If overall technological literacy is not improved, particularly among the technological have-nots, we can expect to see the growth of a "technological divide" more pervasive than today's digital divide. Interesting, well-paying jobs that require a technological understanding and skills will go mostly to well-educated upper- and middle-class Americans and foreign nationals, while the American underclass will continue to be stuck in low-wage, low-skill jobs. On a deeper level, the needs and views of this underclass will, for the most part, not be taken into account by those responsible for developing and setting policy about technology. Thus, new technologies and new applications of existing technologies will be

> Access to a personal computer is the single most important factor in whether or not a person uses the Internet.

largely irrelevant to this group, who will fall further and further outside the mainstream.

Enhancing Social Well-being

It has become a cliché that only the young are up to date on technology, particularly in the fast-moving world of computers and the Internet. Can't figure out how to set up your Web page? Ask a 15-year-old. Confused by e-mail? To many elementary school children it is easier to use than the U.S. mail. But behind the cliché is a basic truth. Technology is changing so rapidly that people who are not prepared to deal with it can quickly find themselves falling behind.

Losing touch in this way can leave people with a sense that they have somehow lost control of their lives, that the world is moving on without them. For much of human history, this was not a problem because changes occurred slowly enough that people had plenty of time to adapt and get used to them. But eras of rapid change—the Industrial Revolution in England, for example, or the United States in the late 1800s and early 1900s—have tested the limits of human adaptability. In times of rapid change, many people struggle to adjust to a world that is suddenly quite different from the one they have known. Even for people who can cope with specific how-tos of modern life, living in a highly technological world can be alienating. This idea has been studied by sociologists and historians and explored in the popular media, including books, movies, and television programs.

> Technological literacy can provide a tool for dealing with rapid changes.

In the next few decades, people's abilities to adjust to new ways of doing things will be tested far more than they have ever been tested before. People in their forties and fifties already often feel as if technology is passing them by; in another generation, people in their thirties could feel the same way. The more adaptable people—those who are invigorated, or at least not threatened, by the new and the unfamiliar—will do well. But many people will find that their sense of well-being and their quality of life are diminished rather than enhanced by new and improved technologies. They will wish that the world were not moving quite as quickly toward the future.

Technological literacy can provide a tool for dealing with rapid changes. A technologically literate person will find it easier to understand and assimilate new technologies and so will be less likely to be left behind.

Equally important, technologically literate people will have a high enough comfort level with and broad comprehension of technology to put the changes in context and accept them even if they do not fully understand them. Technological literacy, along with many other types of literacy, can empower people by giving them the tools to make sense of their world, even as it changes around them.

Conclusion

Much would be gained, for individuals and the country as a whole, by raising the general level of technological literacy in the United States. Of course, even if technological literacy reaches a high level among a majority of Americans, it will not solve all of our problems or compensate for the shortcomings of human nature. There will never be such a panacea. But it seems equally certain that technological literacy will be an essential ingredient to realizing the benefits outlined in this chapter.

A technologically literate public will undoubtedly make some poor decisions. But many more decisions will be good ones that benefit the whole society rather than only one part of it. Participation in itself is no guarantee of sound decision making. But if participation occurs in an environment in which education about technology is common and in which taking part in technological affairs is encouraged, then it will have a positive influence.

Technological literacy in the workplace is likely to be most relevant in technology-intensive industries, such as communications, biotechnology, and aerospace. But employers in other sectors of the economy that are not involved directly in the creation of technology will also reap the benefits. They, too, need employees with basic technological competence and the ability to solve problems. The positive effect of technological literacy on the national economy is necessarily speculative. The arguments that have been made about the importance of literacy in mathematics and science to the economic future of the country are at least as salient in the context of technological literacy.

The case for technological literacy related to the digital divide and social well-being is at heart about equity, about leaving no one behind. Technological literacy is not a sufficient condition for eliminating all inequities, but it is among the necessary conditions for improvement in a modern society.

References

Committee on Workforce Needs in Information Technology. 2001. Building a Workforce for the Information Economy. National Research Council. Washington, D.C.: National Academy Press.

Dalmotas, D.J., J. Hurley, A. German, and K. Digges. 1996. Air bag deployment crashes in Canada. Paper 96-S1O-05, 15th Enhanced Safety of Vehicles Conference, Melbourne, Australia, May 13-17, 1996.

DOC (U.S. Department of Commerce). 2000. Falling Through the Net: Toward Digital Inclusion. Available online at: <http://www.ntia.doc.gov/ntiahome/fttn00/contents00.html> (November 13, 2001).

DOD (U.S. Department of Defense). 2001. Armed Forces Strength Figures for April 2001. Available online at <http://web1.whs.osd.mil/mmid/military/ms0.pdf> (June 26, 2001).

DOL (U.S. Department of Labor). 1991. What Work Requires of Schools: A SCANS Report for America 2000. Washington, D.C.: U.S. Department of Labor.

DOL. 1999. Futurework: Trends and Challenges for Work in the 21st Century. U.S. Department of Labor, Washington, D.C. Available online at: <http://www.dol.gov/asp/futurework/report.htm> (November 13, 2001).

Evans, L. 1991. Traffic Safety and the Driver. New York: Van Nostrand.

Federal Register. 1977. Federal Motor Vehicle Standards: Occupant Protection Systems. 42 (128): 34289–34305.

GAO (General Accounting Office). 2001a. Vehicle Safety: Technologies, Challenges, and Research and Development Expenditures for Advanced Air Bags. Report to the Chairman and Ranking Minority Members, Committee on Commerce, Science, and Transportation, U.S. Senate. June 2001. Washington, D.C.: GAO.

GAO. 2001b. International Trade: Concerns Over Biotechnology Challenge U.S. Agricultural Exports. Report to the Ranking Minority Member, Committee on Finance, U.S. Senate. GAO-01-727. June 2001. Washington, D.C.: GAO.

Hughes, T.P. 1998. Coping with complexity: Central Artery/Tunnel. Pp. 197–254 in Rescuing Prometheus. New York: Pantheon Books.

Laget, P., and M. Cantley. 2001. European responses to biotechnology: Research, regulation, and dialogue. Issues in Science and Technology. Summer 2001. Available online at: <http://www.nap.edu/issues/17.4/p_laget.htm> (December 14, 2001).

NHTSA (National Highway Traffic Safety Administration). 1996. Effectiveness of Occupant Protection Systems and Their Use. Third Report to Congress. Available online at: <http://www.nhtsa.dot.gov/people/injury/airbags/208con2e.html> (November 13, 2001).

Rausch, L.M. 1998. High-Tech Industries Drive Global Economic Activity. Available online at: <http://www.nsf.gov/sbe/srs/issuebrf/sib98319.htm> (November 13, 2001).

21st Century Workforce Commission. 2000. A Nation of Opportunity: Building America's 21st Century Workforce. Washington, D.C.: U.S. Department of Labor.

3
Context for
Technological Literacy

A review of the social, political, and educational context for technological literacy can reveal the opportunities for as well as the obstacles that stand in the way of achieving it. For instance, we can look at the historical role of technology—how technology has changed and how our relationship to it has changed over time. Another factor is people's ideas about technology, specifically, whether or not they have a broad conception of technology consistent with technological literacy. We must also consider the influence of K-12 schooling to determine if students are being afforded an opportunity to develop the three dimensions of technological literacy. In the political arena, we might ask if policy makers have made technological literacy a priority and how they approach technological decisions. We must also try to determine what people actually know about technology and how it is developed.

The Human Connection to Technology

Five hundred years ago, when Europeans first explored the New World, they crossed the sea in wind-powered ships, rode the trail in horse-drawn wagons, and carried muskets for hunting and protection. From our point of view, these technologies were quite simple and easy to comprehend. Although only people with special training knew how to build a ship or sail one, almost everyone could understand what a ship did and how and why. Three centuries later, when the newly established United States was looking westward toward Louisiana and the Pacific, the technologies in use were substantially the same. Although improvements and refinements had been made, a time traveler from 1500 would have had little difficulty adapting to the devices and tools of 1800.

Fast forward another hundred years, however, and it is a different story. By the end of the nineteenth century, a panoply of new technologies had appeared that were qualitatively different from earlier technologies: steamboats and ironclad ships, the telegraph and telephone, the transcontinental railroad, the phonograph, the internal combustion engine, gasoline and other petrochemicals, aspirin and a wealth of other drugs, the automobile, and the machine gun. The world of 1900 was much more dependent upon these machines and tools, which posed challenges that were entirely new. A competent, contributing member of society had to understand and use an increasing number of technological devices.

That pattern continued and accelerated throughout the twentieth century. Today, technology and technological systems are integral to everything we do and can do (Box 3-1). Our homes, our food and water, our jobs, our travel, our communications, our entertainment, our national security are all made possible by and depend on technology.

At the same time that technology has become ubiquitous, people

> By the end of the nineteenth century, a panoply of new technologies had appeared that were qualitatively different from earlier technologies.

BOX 3-1 The Naked City

Technology is so woven into the fabric of modern life that it has become all but invisible. People look at it without seeing it. But try this thought experiment. Take a large city and remove everything provided by technology. What is left?

The buildings are gone, along with their electrical, plumbing, and ventilation systems, phone lines and phones, computers, televisions, furniture, appliances, and every other manufactured product.

All food is gone and all water, except the puddles still standing from last night's rain. The air is still there, but it is noticeably fresher without the gasoline and diesel exhaust, fumes from paints, cleaners, and other volatile liquids, and all particulate matter produced by industrial activity.

Cars and trucks, buses and trains, bicycles and baby carriages are gone. Roads, bridges, tunnels, airports, and other components of our transportation infrastructure—gone. The grass, as natural as it seems, has been grown from seed or sod produced on grass farms, so it too is gone. The weeds remain, but most of the trees, bushes, and flowers, which were raised in nurseries and transplanted, are gone.

Dogs and cats, bred over millennia for specialized traits—gone. The rats and pigeons, which have also been shaped by human activity, but in this case inadvertently, remain, along with insects, squirrels, and other creatures that live alongside humans but are not bred by humans.

Shoes and clothing are gone. So are briefcases, purses, wallets, watches, glasses, contact lenses, hearing aids, wheelchairs, prosthetic devices, heart valves, pacemakers, artificial joints, and all drugs and medicines, both legal and illegal. Any semblance of a health care system—from physicians and nurses to hospitals and ambulances—vanishes. In fact, if it were not for medical technology, many people would also be gone. And of the remaining few, not many would survive for more than a few weeks without the products of human innovation.

have become less and less interested in or able to look below the surface of technology. The reasons for this are easy to find. One important factor is the increasing complexity of technology, which makes it difficult for anyone but experts to work with or understand the technological devices and systems in use today. Two hundred years ago, the family vehicle was a horse-drawn wagon, which was simple and straightforward enough that anyone who examined it could easily understand how it worked. Today the family car is so complicated that parts of it can only be analyzed and serviced with the aid of computerized diagnostic equipment and other specialized devices. Faced with this complexity, many people no longer try to understand how technology works. Instead, we must be content simply learning how to make it do what we want it to. Even specialists who deal with certain technologies—auto mechanics, for instance, or computer technicians—must rely on other technologies they may or may not understand.

Most modern technologies are designed so users do not have to know how they work in order to operate them. We get into our cars, turn the key, put them into drive, and step on the gas without any awareness of the computer-controlled fuel-injection system or the antilock brakes. We click on an icon to retrieve our e-mail with no thought of the complex hardware and software necessary to perform that task. This is hardly surprising; we would get very little done each day if we had to think about the details of our technological helpers before putting them to work.

As technology has become more complex, society has become more specialized. As a result, all of us know more but about fewer things. We turn to plumbers, electricians, appliance repairmen, cable TV install-ers, telephone workers, and other specialists to service or repair our tech-nological devices for the simple reason that we don't have time to learn everything we need to know to take care of them. A doctor or a lawyer or a secretary or a bus driver each has specialized knowledge, but even they tend to learn only as much about technology as they need to do their jobs and, perhaps, to maintain a minimal level of technical competence in their personal lives.

As technology has become more complex, society has become more specialized.

Several other factors have contributed to the lack of hands-on experience with technology. When Americans lived on the farm, they were closely involved with the technologies they used. In general, as the population has shifted from rural to urban and suburban areas, people have become less technologically self-sufficient. In the workplace, in-creasing computerization and automation have made it possible for fewer workers to control more machines, thus reducing the number of people who actually work with machines. At the same time, many jobs have shifted to the service sector, which now accounts for nearly 80 percent of the gross domestic product and a little more than 80 percent of jobs (DOC, 2001). The technical knowledge and capability required of workers in those sectors of the economy that still rely on technically trained people—such as defense, aerospace, and manufacturing—has increased significantly (BLS, 1999). Many employers in these sectors cannot find enough well-trained technicians and have had to invest substantial resources in retraining the people they hire or hire people from abroad (NSF, 1994).

Misconceptions About the Nature of Technology

The nature of technology has changed dramatically in the past hundred years. Indeed, the very idea of technology as we now conceive it is relatively new. For most of human history, technology was mainly the province of craftsmen who passed their know-how down from generation to generation, gradually improving designs and adding new techniques and materials. At the beginning of the Scientific Revolution in the mid-1500s, inventors began using a more rational, rigorous approach to the development of new products and began to apply insights from the physical sciences (Bernal, 1971). Nevertheless, technology remained mostly a trial-and-error discipline. As recently as the late 1800s, most technological progress was made by professional inventors, such as Nikola Tesla, Thomas Edison, and Alexander Graham Bell.

Toward the end of the nineteenth century, a new approach to technology appeared, exemplified by Charles Proteus Steinmetz, who shaped the new field of electricity generation begun by Edison (Hughes, 1983). Unlike Edison, who was an inventor, Steinmetz was an electrical engineer. Instead of relying on intuition and trial and error, he and others like him used detailed calculations based on the latest scientific understanding. They laid out quantitative rules to guide their designs and those of others. Although trial and error was—and still is—an important aspect of technological innovation, the process of engineering design and development has become increasingly systematic and professionalized.

This change, combined with other trends, transformed technology—indeed, created technology as we know it today. By the beginning of the twentieth century, technology had become a large-scale enterprise that depended on large stores of knowledge and know-how, too much for any one person to master. Large organizations were now required for the development, manufacture, and operation of new technologies. Complex networks of interdependent technologies were developed, such as the suite of technologies for the automobile. These include gas and oil refineries, filling stations and repair shops, tire manufacturers, automobile assembly plants, the highway system, and many more. The government began to play a larger role in shaping technology through technological policies and regulations.

The meaning of the word "technology" evolved to reflect these changes (Winner, 1977). In the nineteenth century, technology referred simply to the practical arts used to create physical products, everything from wagon wheels and cotton cloth to telephones and steam engines. In the twentieth century, the meaning of the word was expanded to include everything involved in satisfying human material needs and wants, from factories and the organizations that operate them to scientific knowledge, engineering know-how, and technological products themselves.

As the definition of technology changed, its meaning became more vague, leaving room for misconceptions that sometimes led to questionable conclusions. One widely held misconception relates to how we perceive the relationship among science, engineering, and technology. A second is a technological determinism, a tendency to see technological development as largely independent of human influence.

> By the beginning of the twentieth century, technology had become a large-scale enterprise that depended on large stores of knowledge and know-how, too much for any one person to master.

Technology, Engineering, and Science

Because science has been central to the development of new technologies and the improvement of existing technologies, many people believe that technology is merely the application of science. This idea can be traced to the development of the atomic bomb and radar, two World War II projects in which scientists donned engineering hats to create major technologies almost from scratch. Both efforts were spearheaded by scientists, primarily physicists (Buderi, 1996; Rhodes, 1986).

However, it takes much more than applied science to create a new technology. Technology is a product and a process involving both science and engineering, and the goals of these two disciplines are different. Science aims to understand the "why" and "how" of nature, engineering seeks to shape the natural world to meet human needs and wants.

Engineering, therefore, could be called "design under constraint," with science—the laws of nature—being one of a number of limiting factors engineers must take into account (Wulf, 1998). Other constraints include cost, reliability, safety, environmental impact, ease of use, available human and material resources, manufacturability, government regulations, laws, and even politics. In short, technology necessarily involves science *and* engineering.

In public discourse, innovations and events that have a significant technological component are often described as science.

Yet in public discourse, innovations and events that have a significant technological component are often described as science. Take the building and launching of the Hubble Space Telescope. Although its purpose is scientific—to gather data about the universe and its origins—the telescope itself is the product of science and engineering. Similarly, the development of new drugs is often misidentified solely as science. Obviously, a great deal of scientific research underlies the development of a new drug, but that research is put to work toward a technological end. Even in the computer industry—the first thing that comes to many people's minds when they think of technology—cramming more transistors onto a chip or more memory onto a magnetic disk is a technological, rather than a scientific, advance.

It is not surprising that many people attribute technological advances exclusively to science. After all, as was noted in Chapter 1, science and technology are closely related. But the confusion is significant because it indicates that many people do not appreciate the *combined* role of science, engineering, and technology in shaping modern life. A sense of this complementary relationship is crucial to many policy decisions, for example how public research dollars should be allocated.

Technological Determinism

Another prevalent misconception is that technological change is somehow disconnected from human influence. Technology seems to appear "out of the blue" with little if any input from its intended users. Technology has a dramatic, direct, but one-way effect on our lives. In other words, technology affects society, but society does not affect technology. This idea, sometimes called technological determinism, suggests that technology follows its own course independent of human direction (Smith and Marx, 1994; Winner, 1977).

Technological determinism is based on a misperception of the central role people play in the design and uses of technology. Members of

Congress, company CEOs and the scientists and engineers who work for them, and the consuming public all have a say in what technology should do, what it is capable of doing, and what it actually does. Technology mirrors our values, as well as our flaws. It is merely an agglomeration of parts until we imbue it with purpose and direction (Lafollette and Stine, 1991; Winner, 1977).

If we perceive technology through the lens of technological determinism, we cannot weigh the risks or costs associated with a technology or its benefits. Certain technologies are used in ways that some people find objectionable or that result in unintended and sometimes undesirable consequences (Postman, 1993; Tenner, 1996). And almost always, technologies are more advantageous for some people, animals, plants, generations, or purposes than others. If one views technology as being outside human control, these considerations may never come up.

Thoughtful consideration of possible advantages and disadvantages is extremely important, therefore, *before* a technology is developed. At the same time, we must recognize that perfectly sensible uses of a technology can sometimes have undesirable consequences and that these may not show up for decades or even longer. We may decide, therefore, that not every possible technological advance—human cloning, for example—should be pursued. Or, conversely, we may decide a technology should be developed for the greater good, even though a vocal minority opposes it. In either case, the decision is ours!

Technological Studies in K-12

Developing technological literacy will require early and regular contact with technology in the school setting. Unfortunately, technology has not been the focus of study in K-12 in the United States.

Only 14 states require some form of technology education, usually affiliated with career or technical preparation, for K-12 students (Newberry, 2001). The Massachusetts Board of Education recently added a combined engineering/technology component to its K-12 curriculum, becoming the first state to explicitly include engineering content (*Boston Herald*, December 20, 2000). Elsewhere in the country, the availability of technological studies in grades K-12 varies widely, depending on the school district. A few schools offer stand-alone courses in all grade levels, but most school districts pay little or no attention to it. This is in stark contrast to the situation in some other nations, such as the Czech Repub-

> Almost always, technologies are more advantageous for some people, animals, plants, generations, or purposes than others.

lic, France, Italy, Japan, the Netherlands, Taiwan, and the United Kingdom, where technology education courses are required in middle school or high school (ITEA, unpublished).

Technology education is a relatively new academic subject with roots in the industrial arts movement that began in the early twentieth century. Industrial arts education was intended to develop the skills, including an adeptness with tools, that students would need for jobs in industry. For many students, these classes were purely avocational or recreational.

As metalworking, woodworking, and other shop classes came to seem less and less relevant in the second half of the twentieth century, some industrial arts teachers began to broaden the scope of their classes to include general information about technology—the basic characteristics of a technology, the engineering design process, and how technology shapes society. Although some curricula now include separate classes in technology, many teachers and school officials still think of it as a vocational rather than academic subject (Rogers, 1995). This idea has been reinforced by the longstanding perception that vocational and technology classes—and the students enrolled in them—are of lower status than college-preparatory classes (Gray et al., 1995).

A recent survey of technology education programs in the United States reveals a number of trends, including a shift from the development of tool-related skills to the development of problem-solving abilities, a greater emphasis on the application of science and mathematics, and greater involvement by female faculty and students (Sanders, 2001). A significant minority (40 percent) of technology education programs is still identified most closely with vocational education rather than general education. Many of these programs are, in fact, funded by the Carl D. Perkins Vocational and Technical Education Act of 1998 (P.L. 105-332).

A second limiting factor is the small number of teachers trained to teach about technology. There are roughly 40,000 technology education teachers in the United States, mostly at the middle school or high school level (Newberry, 2001; Weston, 1997). By comparison, about 1.7 million teachers in U.S. K-12 schools (including all elementary school teachers and roughly 150,000 secondary science teachers) are responsible for teaching science (NCES, 2000). Survey data suggest that the percentage of technology teacher positions that goes unfilled is greater than that for the overall teacher workforce (Litowitz, 1998; Weston, 1997). Fewer than 80 programs in the United States are granting degrees in technology education (ITEA, 2001).

A third limiting factor is inadequate preparation of other teachers to teach about technology. Schools of education spend virtually no time developing technological literacy in those who will eventually stand in front of the classroom. As noted elsewhere in this report, the integration of technology content into other subject areas, such as science, mathematics, social studies, English, and art, could greatly boost technological literacy. Without teachers trained to carry out this integration, however, technology is likely to remain an afterthought in American education. The Institute of Electrical and Electronics Engineers (IEEE) is attempting to address this problem by encouraging a dialogue between academic leaders in engineering and education. As a first step, IEEE convened a group of engineering and education school deans in October 2001 to discuss ways to enhance teacher preparation.

> Schools of education spend virtually no time developing technological literacy in those who will eventually stand in front of the classroom.

The paucity of technological studies in mainstream education in the United States is reflected on standardized tests in the traditional areas, such as reading, writing, and math. For example, the Third International Math and Science Study, an ambitious attempt to assess students' understanding of science and math concepts, included virtually no questions related to the understanding, application, or history of technology. Neither the National Assessment of Educational Progress, a test that tracks changes in knowledge in a number of areas, nor the two major college entrance examinations, the SAT and ACT, tests student knowledge of technological concepts, history, or processes.

Because school performance and opportunities for postsecondary education are based largely on these test scores, few administrators are interested in introducing a new subject that does not appear on the standardized tests into the curriculum. Unfortunately, this can prolong the problem. Questions about technology are not likely to be included on standardized tests until technology education is either made a standard school subject or technology content is integrated into other subject areas.

A beginning has been made, however. K-12 students are sometimes introduced to technological concepts through other subject areas, especially science. The two sets of national K-12 science standards developed in the 1990s include specific benchmarks related to technology and design, and a small number of rigorously developed instructional materials that reinforce connections between science and technology have been developed (AAAS, 1993; NRC, 1996); but they are used in only a small percentage of schools.

Ironically, although many so-called hands-on science experiments engage students in technology-related experiences rather than scientific ones, they are not identified as such by either students or teachers. A classic example of this is the "egg-drop" challenge, an exercise in which students are asked to devise a container that can keep an egg from breaking when it is dropped from a certain height. Although the experiment illustrates science concepts, such as momentum and force, teachers usually stress the design, materials, and problem-solving elements of the exercise.

Technological concepts are also addressed in K-12 standards for mathematics, history, language arts, geography, visual arts, civics, economics, health, and behavioral studies (Mid-Continent Research for Education and Learning, 2000). And the standards promulgated by the Council for Basic Education and the National Center on Education and the Economy for a variety of school subjects—including those related to technology, problem solving, and design—have been combined into single publications (CBE, 1998; National Center on Education and the Economy, 1997). However, with a few exceptions, the technology components of these standards have not been translated into curricula or instructional materials. An analysis of some highly rated high school American history textbooks, for example, found almost no mention of technology (Cole, 1996). Given the extent of technology-related changes in society in the last 100 years, such as dramatically increased lifespan, the omission is striking. In one positive development, the Sloan Foundation has funded a group at the Massachusetts Institute of Technology to develop a college-level U.S. history book that will treat science and technology as central forces in the nation's history.

> An analysis of some highly rated high school American history textbooks found almost no mention of technology.

At the national level, the National Science Foundation (NSF) has been the primary funding source for the development of K-12 instructional materials. Since 1994, NSF's instructional materials division has invested about $29 million in some 62 projects (personal communication, G. Salinger, National Science Foundation, August 2, 2001). The agency's spending on technology-related materials has hovered between about 5 and 11 percent of the total for instructional materials in technology, mathematics, and science. NSF's investment in technology teacher enhancement was about $13 million during the same period, about 2 percent of the total spent on teacher enhancement in any one year.

The National Aeronautics and Space Administration (NASA) has for decades considered technology education equal in importance to mathematics and science education. Along with NSF, NASA was instrumental in providing early encouragement and, later, funding to the International Technology Education Association, which has produced K-12 content standards for the study of technology. Although NASA does not fund extramural curriculum development, it supports a broad array of teacher, student, and curriculum enhancement activities associated with NASA facilities and projects throughout the country (NASA, 2001).

Learning About Technology

Exposure to technological concepts and hands-on, design-related activities in the elementary and secondary grades are the most likely ways to help children acquire the kinds of knowledge, ways of thinking and acting, and capabilities consistent with technological literacy. Unfortunately, there is very little information about how children or adults learn concepts in technology and how, or whether, that learning differs from other types of cognition (Cheek, 2000). Much of what is known about how people learn comes from research focused on people with expertise, that is, a combination of conceptual knowledge and procedural knowledge accumulated over time (NRC, 1999b). Studies of engineers and engineering students have focused on two areas of learning relevant to technological literacy: problem solving and design.

Problem Solving. Successful problem solving in engineering or technology education requires both the exercise of knowledge specific to the problem at hand and knowledge that transcends the particular problem or even the discipline.

Hegarty (1991), for example, in a study of knowledge of mechanics, showed that solving real problems with mechanics requires very complex cognitive processes. The choice of a suitable mental model, or problem schema, requires considerable conceptual and procedural knowledge, some of which cannot be easily explained.

Tain-Fung et al. (1996) tested general and technological problem-solving skills in college students pursuing humanities, engineering, and computer science degrees and found no differences in terms of general problem-solving skills. On the technological problem-solving test, however, the computer science students, followed by the engineering students, had the highest test scores. Cooperative learning and problem

There is very little information about how children or adults learn concepts in technology and how, or whether, that learning differs from other types of cognition.

solving are typical elements of technology education, and both have been shown to improve the retention and assimilation of knowledge in a variety of engineering education contexts (Bernold et al., 2000; Catalano and Catalano, 1999; Demetry and Groccia, 1997; Hoit and Ohland, 1998).

Design. Design is a central component of the practice of engineering and a key element in technology education. Good design reflects the designer's tacit knowledge of materials, artifacts, and systems as they relate to one another. The design activities that have been introduced into K-12 technology education in the United States are based on design and technology syllabi and associated curriculum materials developed in Great Britain. So-called design briefs that lay out the functional requirements for a technological design are being introduced into K-12 technology education. Many articles, even in research journals in the field of technology education, strongly advocate the use of design briefs in the school curriculum but do not provide empirical evidence of their effectiveness.

To address these issues, the American Association for the Advancement of Science has begun working with educators in a variety of disciplines to define a research agenda focused on how people learn about technology (AAAS, 2000). The project, which is funded by NSF, is also exploring the most effective methods for teaching technology.

Overemphasis on Computers and Information Technology

The one exception to the general weakness of technological studies in grades K-12 is in the area of computers and information technology. Schools across the country have spent large amounts of money on computers, computer networks, and the Internet, much of it for educational technology—that is, computers and other technological devices used as aids in teaching, practice work, and testing. Only one unit in the U.S. Department of Education, the Office of Educational Technology, promotes the use of technology as a teaching tool, but not the teaching of technology. Since the launch of the Technology Literacy Challenge in 1996, the federal government has invested more than $2 billion[1] in

---

[1]This figure includes spending on Technology Innovation Challenge Grants, the Technology Literacy Challenge Fund, Preparing Tomorrow's Leaders to Use Technology, and Community Technology Centers. It does not include the nearly $5.7 billion collected from consumers by U.S. telecommunications companies to support school and library access to the Internet (through the so-called e-rate program).

programs to increase the use of educational technology in U.S. classrooms (DoEd, 2000).

Many people, even people in the educational system, confuse educational technology with technology education, but the two are quite different. The purpose of technology education is to teach students about technology, while the purpose of educational technology is to use technology to help students learn more about whatever subject they are studying. The other purpose of having computers in schools is to teach students to use computer technologies, from running programs and sending e-mail to setting up websites and surfing the Internet. A number of high-profile reports in the past several years have reinforced the notion that technological literacy is mostly or entirely concerned with the development of computer-related skills (e.g., PCAST, 1997; 21st Century Workforce Commission, 2000). Some limited efforts are also being made to expand the notion of computer literacy to include a basic understanding of the associated hardware and software (Associated Colleges of the South, 2001; NRC, 1999a).

One might suppose that any sort of technology education in the schools, even if it is restricted to computers and information technology, would make it easier to gain acceptance for other sorts of technology education, but the reality is that the use of "technology education" to mean learning about computers and of "technological literacy" to mean facility with computers confuses the issue and leads people to believe that "technology" means little more than computers and related devices. Thus, many people believe that their schools already teach about technology, when in reality they teach only about computers.

A Policy Blind Spot

For the most part, U.S. policy making has rarely addressed the issue of technological literacy. Excluding legislation focused on the use of computers as educational tools, only a handful of bills introduced in Congress in the past 15 years refer to technology education or technological literacy. Virtually none of these bills has become law, except for measures related to vocational education. Three education reform bills were introduced in 2000 by Rep. Vern Ehlers (R-Mich.), one of the two members of Congress who is a physicist. The bills were focused mostly on science and mathematics education but also included provisions that would have strengthened the training of technology teachers and provided

> Many people, even people in the educational system, confuse educational technology with technology education, but the two are quite different.

incentives for schools to hire them. The bills did not reach the floor in the 2000 legislative session, but Ehlers reintroduced them at the beginning of the next Congress. In the same session, House Science Committee Chairman Sherwood L. Boehlert (R-N.Y.) proposed legislation that would, among other things, establish partnerships for enhancing elementary and secondary science and mathematics education. The bill is focused on science and mathematics, but several of the provisions make reference to technology education.

The relative absence of legislative attention to the issue of technological literacy is striking considering the number of issues with a technological component that come before Congress. An unscientific sampling of bills that made it to the president's desk during the 106th Congress reveals the great variety of topics for which an understanding of science and technology would have been useful (Table 3-1). Only 24 members, or slightly more than 4 percent, of the 107th Congress have educational backgrounds in medicine, science, or engineering (AMA, 2001; ASME, 2001).

Of course, Congress does not act in a vacuum. Members can call on the services of the Congressional Research Service, a branch of the Library of Congress, for research on specific topics. Lobbyists, many of whom represent the interests of technology-based industries, are another source of potentially valuable information for congressional decision makers. Members and their staffs also rely on think tanks, such as RAND and MITRE, and advocacy organizations that conduct policy studies, like the Natural Resources Defense Council, for information. Congress and the executive branch often call on the National Academies to examine technical and policy issues in the sciences, engineering, and medicine.

For more than two decades, the congressional Office of Technology Assessment (OTA) was an important source of in-house advice on technological matters. OTA conducted nonpartisan studies of the impacts and possible future directions of technology development. The office was abolished by Congress in 1995. Rep. Rush Holt (D-N.J.), the other physicist in Congress, and a bipartisan group of about 30 representatives sponsored legislation (H.R. 2148) midway through the 107th Congress that would reestablish OTA.

At the state level, lawmakers appear to be slightly more aware of technology education as a school subject. A keyword search of bills under consideration by the states from 1996 to 1999 identified 46 that contained the words "technology" and "education" or the phrase "technological

> The relative absence of legislative attention to the issue of technological literacy is striking considering the number of issues with a technological component that come before Congress.

TABLE 3-1 Technology-Related Bills Approved by the 106th Congress *

Title (Public Law Number)	Technology Provisions (funding level if relevant)
Department of Transportation Appropriations (P.L. 106-69)	Supports development of next-generation, high-speed rail ($27 million appropriated)
Federal Aviation Administration Authorization (P.L. 106-181)	Supports system security technology projects and activities ($53 million authorized) Supports aircraft safety technology projects ($44 million authorized)
National Aeronautics and Space Administration Authorization Act of 2000 (P.L. 106-391)	Provides safety and performance upgrades for the International Space Station ($492 million authorized)
Fire Administration and Earthquake Hazards Reduction Authorizations (P.L. 106-503)	Establishes network for earthquake engineering simulation ($74 million authorized over 4 years)
National Institute of Biomedical Imaging and Bioengineering Establishment Act (P.L. 106-580)	Consolidates dissemination of research, training, and health information across the federal government related to: new imaging techniques and devices; improvements in existing imaging and bioengineering technologies; and technology assessment
Wireless Communications and Public Safety Act of 1999 (P.L. 106-81)	Encourages establishment of a universal emergency telephone number, including for wireless phones Sets forth rules for using wireless phone location and subscriber information
American Competitiveness in the Twenty-First Century Act of 2000 (P.L. 106-313)	Increases substantially the number of aliens eligible for the H-1B visa program, which provides high-skilled workers to U.S. businesses Mandates a U.S. Department of Commerce review of existing public and private high-tech workforce training programs in the United States Requires that the National Science Foundation study the divergence in access to high technology ("digital divide")
Security Assistance Act of 2000 (P.L. 106-280)	Supports science and technology centers in the independent states of the former Soviet Union ($124 million authorized over 2 years)

*In preparing this table, staff with the National Research Council Office of Congressional and Government Affairs searched a database maintained by Congressional Quarterly of all bills passed by both houses during the 106th Congress that contained one or more of the following keywords: competitiveness, education, infrastructure, national security, energy, engineering. This search resulted in a list of 227 bills. Staff of the National Academy of Engineering selected 50 bills that seemed likely to contain significant technology-related provisions and chose the most relevant for the table.

literacy" (personal communication, D.S. Potestio, National Conference of State Legislatures, October 16, 2000). Half were concerned with the use or purchase of information technology, mostly computers. The other half dealt with the support or creation of technology education, applied technology, or industrial arts programs.

Like their federal counterparts, state-level policy makers also require information and advice about science and technology in order to make sound decisions. As states have assumed increasing responsibility for economic development, environmental protection, transportation, health care, job creation, and education, this advice has become even more important. In an effort to leverage technology for economic growth, for example, more than $400 million was invested by states in 1995 to support public-private technology programs (State Science and Technology Institute, 1996). Since then, the amount has certainly increased greatly.

Like their federal counterparts, state-level policy makers also require information and advice about science and technology in order to make sound decisions.

In the 1970s, through its State Science, Engineering and Technology program, NSF spent more than $5 million to help state legislatures increase their technical capabilities. By the time the program ended in 1981, a number of statehouses had begun to support their own programs to integrate scientific and technical information into the decision-making process. Four of 43 state legislative research agencies that responded to a 1998 survey by the Council of State Governments (1999) indicated that they keep scientists, engineers, or statisticians on staff. The majority of the agencies seek out scientific and technical advice on an ad hoc basis through specialists, task forces, state universities, and interns and fellows.

One study of legislators in 11 states found a great—and mostly unmet—need for reliable technical information (Jones et al., 1996). Partly in response to the need for better technical information, in 1999 the National Conference of State Legislatures established a Center for Technical Information (CTI), a nonpartisan information resource for technology- and engineering-related issues for the nation's 7,500 state legislators. The center ceased operation in early 2001 following an unsuccessful fundraising effort (personal communication, L. Morandi, National Conference of State Legislatures, June 19, 2001).

The need for sound science and technology information in the states is also apparent at the executive-branch level. One study of the role of states in science and technology (S&T) concluded that only a few governors had a single source of advice on the broad range of S&T issues (CCSTG, 1992). The report recommended that every governor designate an S&T advisor and that every state establish an independent S&T

advisory council. Currently, about half of the governors have access to some form of S&T information, either through a formally appointed advisor or advisory group or through an informal arrangement with an individual or organization (personal communication, D. Berglund, State Science & Technology Institute, October 25, 2001).

Thus, although there appears to be a recognition at the federal and state levels of the need for information and advice about technological issues, this concern has not led to a recognition of the value of technological literacy for the population at large.

> Currently, about half of the governors have access to some form of S&T information.

Uncertainties About What We Know

Information about what Americans know about technology is hard to come by. A variety of local, state, national, and even international tests measure what U.S. schoolchildren know about mathematics, science, and American history, but few attempts have been made to assess technological knowledge. Similarly, few efforts have been made to determine what the public at large knows about technology, beyond the area of computers.

Technological Literacy of U.S. Students

One has to go back 12 years to find data that shed any light on U.S. students' attitudes and knowledge about technology. In 1988, researchers at Virginia Polytechnic Institute and State University administered a 100-question survey, the Pupils' Attitude Toward Technology (PATT), to more than 10,000 middle school and high school students in seven states (Bame and Dugger, 1989). More than three-quarters of the students who took part in the study were either taking or had taken a technology education or industrial arts class. Two-thirds of the questions were intended to assess attitudes, and one-third were meant to gauge knowledge of technological concepts. The PATT survey was developed and first used in the Netherlands in 1984. Since then, versions of the PATT survey have been used in more than 25 other countries (Bame et al., 1993).

The U.S. researchers focused on the relationship between certain demographic characteristics and responses to related questions. They found, for instance, that boys were more interested in technology than girls, that students' concepts of technology became increasingly accurate with age, and that in general students had a fairly narrow conception of technology. Certain responses were particularly revealing. For example, in reaction to the statement, "In my opinion, technology is not very old," 35 percent of students agreed, and another 27 percent did not know if it was true or not. When asked to consider the statement, "Technology has always to do with mass production," 30 percent agreed, and 35 percent were unsure. Fifty-four percent of students agreed that, "When I think of technology I mostly think of computers," while 30 percent disagreed. These responses suggest that students had a very narrow conception of technology, associated largely with computers, and had only a limited understanding of technology's influence on human history. The results are disturbing, especially considering that most of the participants in the study had some exposure to formal technology education courses.

No assessments of what U.S. students know about technology have been made since the 1989 PATT study. Given the lack of technology studies in U.S. schools, however, it is reasonable to assume that students know less about the nature and history of technology than they do about other, standard subjects, such as mathematics and science. The poor performance of U.S. middle school and high school students on the Third International Math and Science Study (TIMSS) and the recently completed TIMSS follow-up (TIMSS-R) (Gonzales et al., 2000) suggest student technological knowledge would be even lower.

Technological Literacy of U.S. Adults

Only a handful of attempts have been made to measure knowledge and attitudes about technology in the American adult population—except in the area of computers, where scores of surveys have been done in the past decade (e.g., NPR, 1999.) Recently, the International Technology Education Association (ITEA, in press) commissioned the Gallup Organization to conduct the first-ever public poll in the United States on technological literacy. The poll tested conceptual and practical understanding of technology, as well as opinions about the importance of studying technology. ITEA hopes to repeat the survey periodically and use the results as a rough indicator of how—or whether—the level of technological literacy changes over time.

The results of the poll revealed that most Americans have a very limited view of technology. Asked to name the first thing that occurred to them when they thought of technology, the vast majority, nearly 68

> Given the lack of technology studies in U.S. schools, it is reasonable to assume that students know less about the nature and history of technology than they do about other, standard subjects, such as mathematics and science.

percent, said computers. A distant second (almost 4 percent) was electronics. When respondents were given the choice of defining technology as "computers and the Internet" or more broadly as "changing the natural world to satisfy our needs," nearly two-thirds chose the former. Americans also were confused about the relationship among science, engineering, and technology. About 60 percent agreed that engineering and technology *and* that science and technology "are basically the same thing."

About three-quarters of Americans said they understood and were able to use technology to "some extent" or even to a "great extent," but far fewer correctly answered questions testing their knowledge of how specific technologies actually worked (Table 3-2); the discrepancy suggests that our self-rated understanding is superficial. For instance, only half knew that using a cordless phone in the bathtub poses no risk of electrocution, and only a quarter knew that FM radios operate virtually free of static. A much higher proportion, 82 percent, however, knew that cars operate through a series of explosions in the engine, and 62 percent knew that microwave ovens do not work by heating foods from the outside to the inside.

According to the poll, Americans support the idea that people should understand and have some abilities related to technology, and they have a great interest in knowing how technologies work. They also believe strongly that citizens should have input into technology-related decisions that affect them, such as the location of new roads in their

TABLE 3-2 Responses to Questions about Specific Technologies

True or False Statement (correct answer)	% of Americans Responding Correctly
Using a portable phone while in the bathtub creates the possibility of being electrocuted (false)	53
FM radios operate free of static (true)	26
A car operates through a series of explosions (true)	82
A microwave heats food from the outside to the inside (false)	62

Source: ITEA (in press).

community or the development of genetically modified foods and fuel-efficient cars. Ninety-seven percent said they believed the study of technology, broadly defined, should be part of the school curriculum; two-thirds said it should be integrated in other subjects rather than taught as a separate course.

As part of the biennial *Science and Engineering Indicators* report, the National Science Board (NSB) has attempted to measure changes in public attitudes and understanding about science and technology. Jon Miller and his colleagues at the Chicago Academy of Sciences collected and assessed the data, which were first published in 1972. Miller's group used information from telephone surveys to track interest and knowledge of, and attentiveness to, S&T issues. The surveys were administered only to adults. Recently, Miller moved to Northwestern University, and research related to the public understanding of science for the 2002 *Indicators* volume is being conducted by ORC Macro, which is using a survey design very similar to the one developed by Miller's group. NSB plans to redesign the survey in 2003 (personal communication, M. Pollak, National Science Foundation, June 4, 2001).

The American public is no more informed about science and technology than the public in other countries.

The most recent *Indicators* shows that the public is very interested in but relatively poorly informed about science and technology (NSB, 2000). More than 40 percent of respondents rated themselves as very interested in new scientific discoveries and the use of new inventions and technology. Another 40 to 50 percent said they were moderately interested. By contrast, only 17 percent considered themselves very well informed; 30 percent considered themselves poorly informed.

Research by the Pew Center for the People and the Press paints a mixed picture, with people paying close attention to media reporting on certain high-profile science and technology issues but nearly ignoring others (Box 3-2). Cross-national comparisons show that the American public is slightly more interested and has slightly more positive feelings about science and technology but is no more informed about them than the public in other countries (Miller, 1997; Miller et al., 1997; OECD, 1997).

As might be expected, respondents who considered themselves more informed and more interested in science and technology also were better educated and had greater exposure to education in the sciences and mathematics. However, no attempt was made to determine whether the self-assessments were correct, for example whether those who rated themselves well informed actually were well informed. Another study that

BOX 3-2 Technology in the News

From 1986 to 2000, the Pew Research Center for the People and the Press tracked high-profile news stories in the United States and surveyed members of the public to see how closely they were following those stories. The selection of stories was based on the judgment of center staff about what issues the media have been covering most intensively. Of the 735 high-profile stories identified by the center during that time, 54, or 7 percent, had some connection with technology.

The breakdown of those 54 stories is instructive. Sixteen of them, or nearly a third, were about accidents—plane and train crashes, oil spills, and the explosion on the U.S. aircraft carrier Iowa. Eleven related to the U.S. space program, including news about the space shuttle and space station, deployment of the Hubble Space Telescope, and data glitches with the Mars Polar Lander (the 1986 explosion of the Space Shuttle Challenger was included in this group). There were eight biotechnology stories, including items about the cloning of animals and people, the mapping of the human genome, and the controversy surrounding breast implants. Seven stories dealt with some aspect of global climate change, mostly related to unseasonable weather patterns in the United States. Seven stories focused on computers, most of them about the antitrust battle waged by the U.S. government against Microsoft. Four stories concerned testing, arms reduction, or spying related to nuclear weapons technology, and one described structural damage following the 1989 San Francisco earthquake.

It is interesting to see how attentive members of the public were to the various high-profile stories. Eighty percent of those surveyed told the Pew Center researchers that they had followed the Challenger explosion "very closely," but only 50 percent followed the flight of the space shuttle after the Challenger very closely. Fifty-two percent followed the 1989 Exxon Valdez oil spill and 46 percent followed the 1986 Chernobyl nuclear accident very closely. Only 31 percent of those surveyed followed President Bush's 1991 announcement of major nuclear arms reductions very closely, and 24 percent followed the 1990 deployment of Hubble very closely. Many important technology-related stories were followed only by a small share of the public: 18 percent for computer hacker attacks on Yahoo.com and other Internet sites; 17 percent for the cloning of the sheep Dolly; 16 percent for the mapping of the human genome; 9 percent for the debate over global warming; and 8 percent for NASA's discovery of possible life on Mars in 1996.

Source: Adapted from Pew Research Center for the People and the Press, 2001.

attempted to test this correlation using a survey method similar to Miller's found that many people overestimate their level of knowledge about technology (Welty, 1992).

Many of the survey questions in the NSB *Indicators* report lump science and technology together, making it difficult to tease out public knowledge and attitudes specifically about technology. Of the questions that are specific, nearly all of them had to do with science, scientists, or the scientific method. The report looked carefully at the public understanding of the nature of scientific inquiry but did not focus on the public understanding of the design process, which is to engineering roughly what inquiry is to science.

The Miller group's survey attempted to assess people's knowledge of science and technology by testing their ability to judge the correctness of various statements or to define terms. For example, more than 70 percent knew that the continents are moving slowly about the face of the Earth and that light travels faster than sound. But only 13 percent could define a molecule (up from 9 percent in 1995), and fewer than 45 percent knew that lasers do not work by focusing sound waves. Only 16 percent could define the Internet (up from 13 percent in 1997).

Miller also looked at changes over time in the public attitude toward several controversial technologies—nuclear power, genetic engineering, and space exploration. The assessments focused on perceptions of the balance of risks and benefits but did not test an actual understanding of the technology. For example, according to the 2000 *Indicators* report, 48 percent of Americans believed the benefits of nuclear power outweighed the risks, while 37 percent held the opposite view; 15 percent thought the benefits and risks were equal. Forty-four percent of those interviewed agreed that the benefits of genetic engineering either strongly or slightly outweighed the risks.

Taken together, data from the Gallup, NSB, and Pew surveys strongly suggest a mismatch between what Americans know about technology and their reliance on it. In terms of the three dimensions of technological literacy, most Americans exist in a relatively small "space" defined by a combination of limited knowledge, poorly developed ways of thinking and acting, and low capability regarding technology (Figure 3-1).

> Taken together, data from the Gallup, NSB, and Pew surveys strongly suggest a mismatch between what Americans know about technology and their reliance on it.

Technological Literacy in Other Parts of the World

Several countries outside the United States have used various methods to determine the technological literacy of their school children. During the 1999–2000 school year, for example, researchers in the Canadian province of Saskatchewan gave children a five-hour test of their technological knowledge and abilities. Students answered multiple-choice and open-ended essay questions and took part in hands-on activities (Box 3-3). Technology is integrated into all subjects in the K-12 curriculum in Saskatchewan. One purpose of the assessment was to provide a baseline by which to gauge the success of this integration over time (personal communication, C. Atkinson, Saskatchewan Education, June 19, 2000).

Another group of Canadian researchers, with funding from the Ontario Ministry of Education, developed a sophisticated assessment instrument called Views on Science, Technology, and Society (VOSTS)

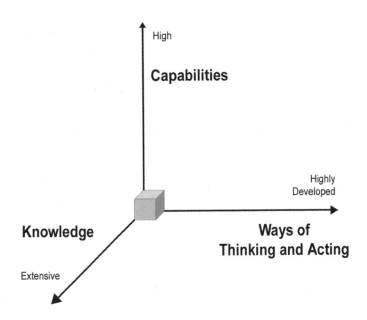

High

Capabilities

Highly
Developed

Knowledge

**Ways of
Thinking and Acting**

Extensive

FIGURE 3-1   The dimensions
of technological literacy,
showing the "space" occupied
by most Americans.

(Crelinsten et al., 1992a). A version of VOSTS has been pilot tested on a cross section of tenth and twelfth grade students but has not been widely administered (Crelinsten et al., 1992b).

In the late 1980s, a research team operating under the auspices of the British School Examinations Assessment Council conducted a large-scale assessment of Britain's design and technology curriculum (Kimbell et al., 1991). The focus of the project, which involved more than 15,000 15-year-olds, was on student performance in design and problem-solving activities rather than on their conceptual understanding of technology. The study concluded that girls generally do better than boys on more reflective design projects and on projects that are loosely defined and that boys do better on projects that require more action and are more tightly bounded.

The European Commission (EC) conducts periodic opinion polls of people in the 17 EC countries to gauge their attitudes, knowledge, and perceptions of risk concerning issues of specific interest to the member governments. Polls that focused on technological topics, mostly biotechnology and genetic engineering, have been published as special reports (e.g., International Research Associates, 2000). A few others were focused on information technology/data privacy and radioactive waste (e.g., International Research Associates, 1997).

The Organisation for Economic Cooperation and Development

BOX 3-3 Testing Conceptions of Technology

What is technology? A telephone? An airplane? What about a cup, a stone axe, a bed? Is a book technology? Is a pair of jeans? A piece of cheese? A flower?

Why do homes use insulation? Why were refrigerators developed? Do all technologies need electricity to operate? Is inventing ways of doing things technology? What is the purpose of having a password when using a computer? What is the most important technology ever made? How did people influence its development? How proficient are you at word processing? How well can you surf the Net? Can you program a clock radio's alarm? Design plans for a new schoolyard? Build a lever from Lego blocks?

If you were a Saskatchewan fifth grader in 1999, you may have had to answer these questions and perform these tasks as part of a wide-ranging assessment of technological literacy. About 1,400 fifth graders and an equal number of 8th and 11th graders in some 187 schools participated in the assessment. Among other things, the results reveal that students have a fairly narrow conception of what technology is. For instance, just 7 percent of 5th and 8th graders, and 18 percent of 11th graders, felt a cup was technology. Similarly small percentages of students identified clothing and musical instruments as technology. Only 31 percent of 11th graders felt an old stone ax was technology. Sixty-two percent of 11th graders and only 23 and 31 percent of 5th and 8th graders, respectively, classed bridges as technology. Fewer than 40 percent of 5th and 8th graders identified a gun as technology, and only two-thirds of 11th graders did so. On the other hand, large majorities in all grades identified electronic technologies (e.g., telephone, computer, microwave oven) as technology.

Source: Saskatchewan Education, 2001.

(OECD) recently initiated the Programme for International Student Assessment (PISA), which measures literacy in reading, mathematics, and science among 15-year-olds in the 29 OECD countries (OECD, 2001). Although the assessment did not explicitly address technological issues, PISA plans to develop an assessment area related to problem solving, which may include technology-related questions (personal communication, S.A. Raizen, National Center for Improving Science Education, May 10, 2001).

Conclusion

The United States finds itself in a paradoxical situation. At this moment, we are the strongest nation in the world economically and militarily, and our strength in both areas depends greatly on technology. In day-to-day affairs, too, we rely—whether we realize it or not—on a vast array of technologies. Under these circumstances, the public and policy makers should place a high value on a basic understanding of technology, including an understanding of how it is created. All Americans should be aware of how technology has shaped our world and should be equipped to make informed choices on issues involving technology.

In reality, the situation is very different. For one thing, as technology has become more sophisticated, more prevalent, and in many cases more "invisible," our human connection to it has changed. In a fundamental way, technology has become unfamiliar to us, not in the sense that we are unable to use it—in fact, Americans are adept consumers and users of technology—but unfamiliar in the deeper sense of not understanding how or why technology is created or what makes it work. Therefore, most Americans have little feel for the limits and potential of technology. This distancing has caused a number of misconceptions to spring up, for example about the relationship among science, engineering, and technology. And it has narrowed our idea of what technology is.

> In a fundamental way, technology has become unfamiliar to us.

The institutions—schools, primarily—with the capability to address this lack of knowledge and these misconceptions have not been called on to do so. Technological studies, whether dedicated technology education courses or integrated as part of other subjects, have been relegated to the back burner of the K-12 agenda. Some important initiatives that could be vital building blocks in addressing this shortcoming have been undertaken (see Chapter 5), but the current situation is discouraging.

Ironically, the one area of technology—computers and the Internet—that has received the attention of both the public and policy makers seems to have further diminished the prospects for technological literacy. The focus on computers has distracted everyone—from students and classroom teachers to business leaders and legislators—from the growing, unmet larger need for an understanding of the nature, history, and role of technology. On Capitol Hill and in statehouses across the country, the issue of technological literacy is rarely discussed. This policy-making blind spot is indeed troubling given the thicket of technological issues lawmakers must negotiate on a daily basis.

The results of the ITEA-commissioned Gallup poll have revealed a deeply rooted problem. Most Americans have a very narrow view of technology. And although many appear to be confident in their ability to manage the complexities of the technological world, they also lack an understanding of how certain common technologies operate. The poll represents only a snapshot of public opinion, of course. Very few data are available about what U.S. students or the public at large actually knows about technology. This lack of information makes it difficult to design and evaluate approaches for boosting technological literacy, either in the school setting or outside of the formal educational system.

Overall, the current context for technological literacy creates more obstacles than opportunities. For reasons that are at once historical, institutional, and reflective of the nature of modern technology, Americans appear to be unprepared to engage effectively and responsibly with technological change. To put it bluntly, we are a nation that does not value technological literacy and, therefore, has not achieved it.

References

AAAS (American Association for the Advancement of Science). 1993. Benchmarks for Science Literacy. New York: Oxford University Press.

AAAS. 2000. Proceedings of the AAAS Technology Education Research Conference. Available online at: <http://www.project2061.org/technology/default.htm> (November 15, 2001).

AMA (American Medical Association). 2001. 2000 Physician Incumbents. Unpublished data assembled by AMA Media office. Washington, D.C.

ASME (American Society of Mechanical Engineers). 2001. Is there an engineer in the House? ASME International Capitol Update. January 17, 2001. Available online at: <http://www.asme.org/gric/Update/2001/011701.html#2> (June 21, 2001).

Associated Colleges of the South. 2001. Information Fluency. Available online at: <http://www.colleges.org/~if/index.html> (November 15, 2001).

Bame, E.A., and W.E. Dugger, Jr. 1989. Pupils' Attitude Toward Technology—PATT-USA Report Findings. Paper. October 25, 1989.

Bame, E.A., W.E. Dugger, Jr., M. deVries, and J. McBee. 1993. Pupils' attitudes toward technology—PATT-USA. Journal of Technology Studies 19(1): 40–48.

Bernal, J.D. 1971. Science in History. Vol. 2: The Scientific and Industrial Revolution. Cambridge, Mass.: MIT Press.

Bernold, L.E., W.L. Bingham, P.D. McDonald, and T.M. Attia. 2000. Impact of holistic and learning-oriented teaching on academic success. Journal of Engineering Education 89(2): 191–199.

BLS (Bureau of Labor Statistics). 1999. Report on the American Workforce. Available online at: <http://stats.bls.gov/opub/rtaw/rtawhome.htm> (November 15, 2001).

Buderi, R. 1996. The Invention that Changed the World: How a Small Group of Radar Pioneers Won the Second World War and Launched a Technological Revolution. New York: Simon & Schuster.

Catalano, G.D., and K. Catalano. 1999. Transformation: from teacher-centered to student-centered engineering education. Journal of Engineering Education 88(1): 59–64.

CBE (Council for Basic Education). 1998. Standards for Excellence in Education—A Guide for Parents, Teachers, and Principals for Evaluating and Implementing Standards for Education. Washington, D.C.: CBE.

CCSTG (Carnegie Commission on Science, Technology, and Government). 1992. Science, Technology, and the States in America's Third Century. New York: CCSTG.

Cheek, D. 2000. Cognitive Science and Technology Education. Background paper prepared for the National Academy of Engineering/National Research Council Committee on Technological Literacy.

Cole, J.R. 1996. The two cultures revisited. The Bridge 26(3–4): 16–21.

Council of State Governments. 1999. A State Official's Guide to Sound Science. Available online at: <http://stars.csg.org/reports/1999/science/menu.htm> (November 15, 2001).

Crelinsten, J., J. de Boerr, and G. Aikenhead. 1992a. Measuring Students' Understanding of Science in Its Technological and Social Context. Volume 1: Designing a Suitable Instrument. Toronto: Queen's Printer for Ontario.

Crelinsten, J., J. de Boerr, and G. Aikenhead. 1992b. Measuring Students' Understanding of Science in Its Technological and Social Context. Volume 2: Validating the Instrument. Toronto: Queen's Printer for Ontario.

Demetry, C., and J.E. Groccia. 1997. A comparative assessment of students' experiences in two instructional formats of an introductory materials science course. Journal of Engineering Education 86(3): 203–210.

DOC (U.S. Department of Commerce). 2001. Economic Report of the President of the Council of Economic Advisors, January 2001. Available online at: <http://w3.access.gpo.gov/usbudget/fy2002/erp.html> (November 15, 2001).

DoEd (U.S. Department of Education). 2000. Progress Report on Educational Technology, State-By-State Profiles, November 2000. Available online at: <http://www.ed.gov/Technology/progress-statebystate-2000.pdf> (November 15, 2001).

Gonzales, P., C. Calsyn, L. Jocelyn, K. Mak, D. Kastberg, S. Arafeh, T. Williams, and W. Tsen. 2000. Pursuing Excellence: Comparisons of International Eighth-Grade Mathematics and Science Achievement from a U.S. Perspective, 1995 and 1999. Washington, D.C.: National Center for Education Statistics.

Gray, K., W.J. Wang, and S. Malizia. 1995. Is vocational education still necessary? Investigating the educational effectiveness of the college prep curriculum. Journal of Industrial Teacher Education 32(2): 6–29. Also available online at: <http://borg.lib.vt.edu/ejournals/JITE/v32n2/gray.html> (November 15, 2001).

Hegarty, M. 1991. Knowledge and processes in mechanical problem solving. Pp. 253–286 in Complex Problem Solving: Principles and Mechanisms, edited by R.J. Sternberg and P.A. Frensch. Hillsdale, N.J.: Lawrence Erlbaum Associates.

Hoit, M., and M. Ohland. 1998. The impact of a discipline-based introduction to engineering course on improving retention. Journal of Engineering Education 87(1): 79–85.

Hughes, T.P. 1983. Networks of Power: Electrification in Western Society, 1880–1930. Baltimore: Johns Hopkins University Press.

International Research Associates. 1997. Eurobarometer 46.1. Information Technology and Data Privacy. Report produced for the European Commission, Directorate General "Internal Market and Financial Services" by INRA (Europe) - E.C.O. January 1997. Brussels: INRA (Europe).

International Research Associates. 2000. Eurobarometer 52.1. The Europeans and Biotechnology. Report by INRA(Europe) - ECOSA on behalf of Directorate-General for Research, Directorate B- Quality of Life and Management of Living Resources Programme. March 15, 2000. Brussels: INRA (Europe).

ITEA (International Technology Education Association). 2001. ITEA Institutional Members Offering Technology Education Degree Programs. Available online at: <http://www.iteawww.org/J4.html> (November 15, 2001).

ITEA. In press. ITEA/Gallup Poll Reveals What People Think About Technology. Reston, Va.: ITEA.

ITEA. Unpublished. Results of 1997 Survey of the Status of Technology Education in 14 Nations.

Jones, M., D.H. Guston, and L.M. Branscomb. 1996. Informed Legislatures: Coping with Science in a Democracy. Lanham, Md.: University Press of America.

Kimbell, R., K. Stables, T. Wheeler, A. Wosniak, and V. Kelly. 1991. The Assessment of Performance in Design and Technology, The Final Report of the APU Design and Technology Project, 1985–1991. London: School Examinations and Assessment Council.

Lafollette, M., and J. Stine. 1991. Contemplating choice: Historical perspectives on innovation and application of technology. Pp. 1–17 in Technology and Choice: Reading from Technology and Culture, edited by M. Lafollette and J. Kline. Chicago: University of Chicago Press.

Litowitz, L.S. 1998. Technology education teacher demand and alternative route licensure. The Technology Teacher 58(5): 23–28.

Mid-Continent Research for Education and Learning. 2000. K-12 Standards—Content Knowledge. Available online at <http://www.mcrel.org/standards-benchmarks/> (November 15, 2001).

Miller, J. 1997. Public Understanding of Science and Technology in OECD Countries: A Comparative Analysis. Paper presented to the 1996 OECD Symposium on Public Understanding of Science and Technology, Tokyo, Japan, November 5, 1996. Revised February 8, 1997.

Miller, J., R. Pardo, and F. Niwa. 1997. Public Perceptions of Science and Technology—A Comparative Study of the European Union, the United States, Japan, and Canada. Bilbao, Spain: BBV Foundation.

NASA (National Aeronautics and Space Administration). 2001. A Guide to NASA Education Programs. Available online at: <http://ehb2.gsfc.nasa.gov/edcats/2000/nep/programs/index.html> (November 15, 2001).

National Center on Education and the Economy. 1997. New Standards. Performance Standards—English Language Arts, Mathematics, Science, Applied Learning. Washington, D.C.: New Standards.

NCES (National Center for Education Statistics). 2000. Digest of Education Statistics, 2000. Available online at: <http://nces.ed.gov/pubs2001/digest/dt068.html> (November 15, 2001).

Newberry, P. 2001. Technology education in the U.S.: a status report. The Technology Teacher 61(1): 8–12.

NPR (National Public Radio). 1999. Survey Shows Widespread Enthusiasm for High Technology—Americans Love Their Computers and the Internet; "Digital Divide" Still Exists, but There Is Good News, Too. Available online at: < http://www.npr.org/programs/specials/poll/technology/> (November 15, 2001).

NRC (National Research Council). 1996. National Science Education Standards. Washington, D.C.: National Academy Press.

NRC. 1999a. How People Learn: Brain, Mind, Experience, and School. Washington, D.C.: National Academy Press.

NRC. 1999b. Being Fluent in Information Technology. Washington, D.C.: National Academy Press.

NSB (National Science Board). 2000. Science and Technology: Public Attitudes and Public Understanding. Chapter 8 in Science and Engineering Indicators 2000—Volume 1. Arlington, Va.: National Science Foundation.

NSF (National Science Foundation). 1994. Gaining the Competitive Edge: Critical Issues in Science and Engineering Technician Education. A Report from a Workshop Sponsored by the National Science Foundation and the Federal Coordinating Council on Science, Engineering, and Technology. July 1993.

Available online at: <http://www.nsf.gov/pubs/stis1994/nsf9432/nsf9432.txt> (November 15, 2001).

OECD (Organisation for Economic Cooperation and Development). 1997. Science and Technology in the Public Eye. Report of a symposium held November 5–6, 1996, in Tokyo, Japan. Paris: OECD.

OECD. 2001. Measuring Student Knowledge and Skills. The PISA 2000 Assessment of Reading, Mathematical, and Scientific Literacy. Available online at: <http://www.oecd.org/els/education/stats.htm> (November 15, 2001).

PCAST (President's Committee of Advisors on Science and Technology). 1997. Report to the President on the Use of Technology to Strengthen K-12 Education in the United States. March 1997. Panel on Educational Technology. Available online at: <http://www.ostp.gov/PCAST/k-12ed.html> (November 21, 2001).

Pew Research Center for the People and the Press. 2001. Public Attentiveness to News stories: 1986–2000. Available online at: <http://www.people-press.org/database.htm> (November 15, 2001).

Postman, N. 1993. Technopoly: The Surrender of Culture to Technology. New York: Vintage Books.

Rhodes, R. 1986. The Making of the Atomic Bomb. New York: Simon & Schuster.

Rogers, G.E. 1995. Technology education curricular content: a trade and industrial education perspective. Journal of Industrial Teacher Education 32(3): 59–74. Also available online at: <http://scholar.lib.vt.edu/ejournals/JITE/v32n3/Rogers.html> (November 15, 2001).

Sanders, M. 2001. New paradigm or old wine? The status of technology education practice in the United States. Journal of Technology Education 12(2): 35–55. Also available online at: <http://scholar.lib.vt.edu/ejournals/JTE/v12n2/sanders.html> (November 15, 2001).

Saskatchewan Education. 2001. 1999 Provincial Learning Assessment in Technological Literacy. May 2001. Available online at: <http://www.sasked.gov.sk.ca/k/pecs/ae/docs/plap/techlit/1999TechLit.pdf> (November 15, 2001).

Smith, M.R., and L. Marx, eds. 1994. Does Technology Drive History: The Dilemma of Technological Determinism. Cambridge: MIT Press.

State Science and Technology Institute. 1996. State Funding for Cooperative Technology Programs, June 1996. Available online at: <http://www.ssti.org/Publications/StateFund_96.pdf> (November 15, 2001).

Tain-Fung, W., R.L. Custer, M.J. Dyrenfurth. 1996. Technological and personal problem solving styles: Is there a difference? Journal of Technology Education 7(2): 55–71.

Tenner, E. 1996. Why Things Bite Back: Technology and the Revenge of Unintended Consequences. New York: Knopf.

21st Century Workforce Commission. 2000. A Nation of Opportunity: Building America's 21st Century Workforce. Washington, D.C.: U.S. Department of Labor.

Welty, K. 1992. Technological literacy and political participation in McLean County, Illinois. Journal of Industrial Teacher Education 29(4): 7–22.

Weston, S. 1997. Teacher shortage—supply and demand. The Technology Teacher 57(2): 6–9.

Winner, L. 1977. Autonomous Technology: Technics-out-of-Control as a Theme in Political Thought. Cambridge, Mass.: MIT Press.

Wulf, W.A. 1998. Diversity in engineering. The Bridge 28(4): 8–13.

4
Foundation for Technological Literacy

I n the past several decades, curriculum developers, engineering professional societies, science centers, and others have devoted effort to initiatives that have improved technological literacy, even if that was not their explicit aim. These span everything from projects to develop instructional materials for the classroom to television programs and museum exhibits. Given the absence of technological literacy on the agendas of both the policy making and education communities in the United States, these initiatives, although modest by comparison with other literacy initiatives, are encouraging. Although the organizations and individuals promoting these initiatives have been working away in relative obscurity, they do constitute a resource for more ambitious efforts.

K-12 Schools

The study of technology in the K-12 classroom has three distinct forms: (1) a theme in other disciplines, especially science; (2) formal technology education classes; and (3) technician-preparation, vocational, and school-to-career programs, which approach technological understanding and skills as means to employment.

Technology as a Theme Within Science and Other Subjects

One of the first attempts to integrate the study of science and technology in the secondary school curriculum was *Man-Made World*, a series of textbooks developed at the State University of New York, Stony Brook, as part of the Engineering Concepts Curriculum Project (1971). Although the texts were never widely adopted, they provided a model for other projects. A decade later, an analysis of studies of science education and student assessments suggested that science education must be focused on content that would prepare students to live and work in a world in which science, technology, and society continually interact (Harms and Yager, 1981). Science textbooks of the day devoted almost no space to the topic of technology or global issues, such as population growth, world hunger, and air quality (Hamm and Adams, 1989; Piel, 1981).

The notion that the social dimensions of science and technology should be part of the science curriculum was echoed in a number of education policy documents of the period (e.g., NCEE, 1982; NSB, 1983; NSTA, 1982). The holistic consideration of subjects that had traditionally been treated separately reflected the growing popularity of the so-called science, technology, and society (STS) paradigm in the United States (Yager, 1996). The influence of these policies on what children were actually taught about technology is difficult to determine. Indirect evidence, such as a 1993 survey of state science supervisors that found that one-third either required or recommended attention to STS themes as part of their science curricula, suggests that STS policies did have an effect, if only by raising expectations (Kumar and Berlin, 1996). Instructional materials, such as the *Innovation* series of the Biological Sciences Curriculum Study (BSCS, 1984), those developed by the school district of Wassau, Wisconsin (Harkness et al., 1986), and modules created by the New York Science, Technology, and Society Education Project, were among the first to carry the STS theme into U.S. classrooms.

In 1989, the American Association for the Advancement of Science (AAAS) published *Science for All Americans*, an elegantly reasoned treatise on the importance of science literacy. The report, and the AAAS standards that followed 4 years later, *Benchmarks for Science Literacy* (1993), emphasized the importance of technology to science and the interrelationship between science, technology, and society. The *National Science Education Standards*, another set of comprehensive science standards developed several years later by the National Research Council (NRC) (1996), reinforced the curricular connections between science and technology. These two sets of science standards were the most detailed descriptions of technological literacy for students until the recent publication of *Standards for Technological Literacy: Content for the Study of Technology* (ITEA, 2000).

Many newer instructional materials have tried to meet one or both sets of science standards. These include BSCS's *Science T.R.A.C.S.* (Teaching Relevant Activities for Concepts and Skills; 2000), which includes a science and technology strand for K-5 students, and *Middle School Science and Technology* (2000), which touches on a variety of technological concepts related to change, diversity, limits, and systems. The Lawrence Hall of Science at the University of California Berkeley, under its Science Education for Public Understanding program, has produced three year-long courses and a number of shorter curriculum modules that touch on technological issues. The National Science Resources Center, jointly operated by the Smithsonian Institution and the National Academies, has produced science materials for elementary students (*Science and Technology for Children*) and is developing materials for use in middle school (*Science and Technology Concepts for Middle Schools*).

A number of NSF-funded projects have developed materials that integrate technology with other subjects, especially mathematics and science (e.g., Integrated Mathematics, Science, and Technology, 2001; Integrating Mathematics, Science, and Technology in the Elementary Schools, 2001). Several of these projects have examined the effects of the technology component on student learning in math and science. In at least one case, scores on international math and science achievement tests were higher among students using the integrated curriculum than in a control group that did not use the materials, suggesting that the technology component of the curriculum boosts learning in other subject areas (Loepp et al., 2000). Similar spin-off benefits in math, science, and reading achievement were found in elementary schools that piloted a curriculum emphasizing contextual learning and design activities (Todd and Hutchinson, 2000).

Some features of technological studies, especially encouraging students to identify and design solutions to problems significant in their own lives, may make other academic subjects more interesting and meaningful. For this reason, technology has been recognized as a topic worthy of study by a variety of disciplines outside of science. For instance, the National Council of Teachers of English (NCTE) has cosponsored many of the annual national technological literacy conferences organized by the National Association for Science, Technology, and Society. Papers presented at this conference have addressed varied topics, such as focusing on

> A number of NSF-funded projects have developed materials that integrate technology with other subjects, especially mathematics and science.

> **BOX 4-1 Whole Cloth: Discovering Science and Technology Through the History of American Textiles**
>
> The Smithsonian Institution's Lemelson Center, in partnership with the Society for the History of Technology and the Education Development Center, has developed eight independent curriculum units that examine the history of textiles, the technology and science of their production, and their consumption. Each unit deals with an aspect of cloth or clothing production or use and includes 5 to 10 exercises, a teacher's essay, and a bibliography. The modules are coordinated with traditional American history, American studies, and American social history courses as taught in middle schools and high schools. Students are asked to interpret primary historical documents, create graphs and charts, and engage in debates and class discussions. The units on early American industrialization, the technology and invention of dyes and dyeing, and the development of nylon, are available online at: <http://www.si.edu/lemelson/centerpieces/whole_cloth/index.html>.

technology, work, and values through poetry (Amram, 1989); improving critical thinking about STS issues through creative writing (Fagan, 1989; Hankins, 1989; Tangum, 1989); and improving student understanding of the complexities of STS issues through drama (Miller and Butcher, 1990). Interesting materials have also been developed combining content from social studies and technology (Box 4-1).

Technology Education

Technology educators are playing an increasingly important role in the development and delivery of technology-related content to students in K-12 classrooms, and technology teachers represent an important resource for attempts to boost U.S. technological literacy. The recent publication of *Standards for Technological Literacy: Content for the Study of Technology* (ITEA, 2000) establishes 20 standards in five categories to guide curriculum development for all K-12 students (Box 4-2). ITEA is in the process of developing standards for teacher development, student assessment, and program development to provide a comprehensive vision of technological literacy in a school setting.

During the 7-year process of developing the standards, ITEA worked closely with a number of other organizations that had previously had little if any connection to the technology education community. These organizations included national associations representing math and science teachers, the AAAS, and the National Academies. ITEA benefited

BOX 4-2   ITEA Standards for Technological Literacy

Nature of Technology

Standard 1   Students will develop an understanding of the characteristics and scope of technology.

Standard 2   Students will develop an understanding of the core concepts of technology.

Standard 3   Students will develop an understanding of the relationships among technologies and the connections between technology and other fields of study.

Technology and Society

Standard 4   Students will develop an understanding of the cultural, social, economic, and political effects of technology.

Standard 5   Students will develop an understanding of the effects of technology on the environment.

Standard 6   Students will develop an understanding of the role of society in the development and use of technology.

Standard 7   Students will develop an understanding of the influence of technology on history.

Design

Standard 8   Students will develop an understanding of the attributes of design.

Standard 9   Students will develop an understanding of engineering design.

Standard 10   Students will develop an understanding of the role of troubleshooting, research and development, invention and innovation, and experimentation in problem solving.

Abilities for a Technological World

Standard 11   Students will develop abilities to apply the design process.

Standard 12   Students will develop abilities to use and maintain technological products and systems.

Standard 13   Students will develop abilities to assess the impact of products and systems.

The Designed World

Standard 14   Students will develop an understanding of and be able to select and use medical technologies.

Standard 15   Students will develop an understanding of and be able to select and use agricultural and related biotechnologies.

Standard 16   Students will develop an understanding of and be able to select and use energy and power technologies.

Standard 17   Students will develop an understanding of and be able to select and use information and communication technologies.

Standard 18   Students will develop an understanding of and be able to select and use transportation technologies.

Standard 19   Students will develop an understanding of and be able to select and use manufacturing technologies.

Standard 20   Students will develop an understanding of and be able to select and use construction technologies.

Source: ITEA, 2000.

from the support of the NSF and the National Aeronautics and Space Administration, which jointly funded the standards project.

Technician-Preparation, Vocational, and School-to-Career Programs

Although technicianpreparation, vocational, and school-to-career programs are mostly intended to prepare people for jobs, they can also enhance some attributes of technological literacy.

Although technological literacy is not the same as technical proficiency, courses and skill development in one area of technology can lead to a better understanding of the nature, history, and role of technology in general. Therefore, although technician-preparation, vocational, and school-to-career programs are mostly intended to prepare people for jobs, they can also enhance some attributes of technological literacy.

Technician Preparation

The Carl D. Perkins Vocational Education Act (P.L. 98-524) enacted by Congress in 1984 stimulated the development of technician-preparation programs. Students in tech prep take courses during their last 2 years of high school that are linked (articulated) with two-year associate degree programs at community colleges (Box 4-3).

A consortium of states, through the Texas-based Center for Occupational Research and Development (CORD), developed many of the first tech-prep courses. CORD curriculum materials were the first to teach physics, chemistry, communications (English language arts), and mathematics in an applied way for students whose career goals might depend on skills developed in a two-year technical program. *Principles of*

BOX 4-3 Technology Studies in Community Colleges

Community colleges play an important part in promoting job-related technological competency by training tens of thousands of people every year in a variety of technology-related fields. According to the National Center for Education Statistics (NCES), a total of 998 private or public two-year institutions offer engineering-related technologies programs. Slightly more than 20,000 individuals graduated with associate degrees in this area in the 1996–1997 school year, making it the fourth most popular community-college program. An additional 6,200 people earned engineering technology certificates that year. By comparison, the 955 programs in computer and information sciences awarded about 8,000 associate degrees in 1996–1997.

Source: NCES, 2000a.

Technology, a two-year, 14-unit, high-school physics curriculum first published in 1984, remains the classic tech-prep textbook (CORD, 1984). The text was recently adapted for a one-year program and reissued as *Physics in Context* (CORD, 2001).

In recent years, the tech prep concept has been expanded at the federal and state levels to embrace students preparing for a wider range of careers. According to NCES, about half of comprehensive U.S. high schools now offer tech-prep courses (NCES, 2000b), and a variety of instructional materials have been developed to meet this demand. For example, *Science in a Technical World*, a set of 12 modules developed with NSF support, is intended for applied science courses in grades 11 and 12. Published by W.H. Freeman, current module topics include the Carbonated Beverage Industry, Wastewater Treatment Industry, Plant Tissue Culture, Paint Research and Development, Petroleum Refining, Petroleum Location, Polymer Research and Development, and Pulp and Paper.

In 1993, NSF initiated the Advanced Technology Education (ATE) program to support curriculum development and program improvement at selected community colleges. Recipients of ATE awards, usually in collaboration with local secondary schools, four-year colleges and universities, and industry, offer students training in many fields, such as biotechnology, computer and information systems, manufacturing technology, and telecommunications. From fiscal year 1994 through fiscal year 2001, NSF invested $222 million in 420 ATE projects (personal communication, G. Salinger, National Science Foundation, August 2, 2001).

Vocational Education

The federal government divides vocational education at the high school level into three categories: (1) courses that prepare students for specific jobs in such areas as agriculture, business, health care, marketing, and trade and industry; (2) courses in family and consumer sciences; and (3) more general courses, such as keyboarding, industrial arts classes, and technology education classes. The trade and industry programs, which include courses in construction, mechanics and repair, and precision production, were the most popular in 1994, the latest year for which data are available. Eight percent of high school students took three or more courses in this area, compared to 16 percent in 1982, reflecting a general decline in student interest in vocational courses and a shift toward college-

> In recent years, the tech-prep concept has been expanded at the federal and state levels to embrace students preparing for a wider range of careers.

prep curricula (NCES, 2000b). In 1994, 97 percent of U.S. high school graduates had taken at least one vocational course, almost the same number as in 1982.

School-to-Career Programs

The 1994 School to Work Opportunities Act (P.L. 103-239) focused on coordinating school-based learning and work-based learning and integrating vocational and academic learning for all students, not just those in vocational programs. Many private companies support school-to-work programs as a way of increasing the pool of qualified entry-level workers and reducing the amount of training business must provide for new workers. All 50 states have received federal funds to develop school-to-work partnerships, and nearly three-quarters have enacted laws to continue the partnerships after the federal program ends in 2001 (National School to Work Office, 2000). The connections between tech prep and the school-to-career movement are still being worked out in each state.

Through the National Skill Standards Board (NSSB), the federal government has also been working to develop skill standards for 15 industry sectors. The standards are being developed by volunteers from business, labor, civil rights, and community groups. Standards in manufacturing and sales and service are almost complete, and standards in the education and training, utility, and hospitality and tourism industries are under development (NSSB, 2000). Industry sectors with strong connections to technology include construction; scientific and technical support; and telecommunications, computers, and arts and entertainment. The NSSB is also compiling information on certification and apprenticeship programs around the country in the 15 industry sectors.

Postsecondary Education

The study of technology during the formative years in the K-12 grades is crucial to the development of technological literacy. A number of opportunities for more advanced study of technology are also available, mostly for people pursuing careers as K-12 teachers, curriculum developers, or scholars. Postsecondary education plays an important role in developing the human infrastructure that can support technological literacy.

Undergraduate and Graduate Science, Technology, and Society Programs

In the late 1960s and early 1970s, a number of colleges and universities launched programs or courses designed to increase student awareness of interactions among science, technology, and society (STS). In 1982, the Alfred P. Sloan Foundation initiated the New Liberal Arts Program, a series of grants to about 30 colleges to help them integrate the study of technology and the engineering process into the general curriculum (Sloan Foundation, press release, November 9, 1982).

The most recent survey to track the progress of STS showed that there were 127 complete programs in 92 American colleges and universities (De la Mothe, 1983). About 100 are estimated to exist today (personal communication, S. Cutcliffe, Lehigh University, December 12, 2000). Even well-established STS programs face substantial hurdles, such as opposition from faculty in traditional disciplines, difficulties in staffing, and maintaining the multidisciplinary approaches STS studies require (Foltz, 1988).

> About 100 STS programs exist in the United States today.

Undergraduate majors in STS have been available for some time at elite colleges and research universities, such as Stanford, Cornell, Pennsylvania State University, University of Pennsylvania, Rensselaer Polytechnic Institute, North Carolina State University, Massachusetts Institute of Technology, and Vassar. Many of the same schools have had graduate programs dealing with technology and society for many years. These programs vary widely in their emphasis on social sciences, history, engineering, and the physical sciences.

Writing and Interdisciplinary Courses in Engineering

Engineering programs have begun to emphasize writing courses in the undergraduate curriculum. One goal of this movement is to ensure that future engineers can convey complex technical concepts and principles to the lay public. These "engineering writing" courses are an example of how the engineering community is attempting to communicate with the larger society, which is affected by the work of engineers.

Since the 1980s and 1990s, many engineering schools have required that all undergraduate engineering students take one or more courses on the social impacts of technology. At Penn State, the largest engineering school in the nation, these courses have been required for all students since the late 1980s. Similar requirements have been adopted by many other institutions, including Worcester Polytechnic, University of Virginia, Stanford, MIT, Lehigh, Cal Tech, and most of the large state-supported engineering schools.

History, Philosophy, and Sociology of Technology Programs

The first formal courses outside of engineering schools dealing with technology were developed by departments of history and the philosophy of science. Scholars in these disciplines generally considered technology "applied science," which is apparent in *Isis*, the official journal of the History of Science Society. The society also publishes *Osiris*, an annual volume of research on the history of science and its cultural influences. History of science programs at the undergraduate and graduate levels have always addressed technology issues. Recently, the Society for the Social Study of Science has applied sociological, anthropological, and sociological techniques to the study of science. The organization's *Handbook of Science and Technology Studies* is a landmark reference work in this arena (Jasanoff et al., 1995).

Historians have written about technology since the late 1800s (Hughes, in press). In 1958, Melvin Kranzberg and other historians of technology founded the Society for the History of Technology (SHOT), signaling that the study of technology should become a formal, recognized discipline separate and distinct from the study of science. The first issue of the society's journal, *Technology and Culture*, featured articles by Lewis Mumford, Peter Drucker, Kranzberg, and others that laid out a vision and research agenda for this new discipline. Today, many colleges and universities offer history, sociology, and philosophy of technology programs, and the research agenda envisioned by Kranzberg and associates has been amplified and fleshed out by symposia, books, and articles. Membership in SHOT now stands at more than 2,000 individuals and 1,500 institutions worldwide (SHOT, 2000).

Philosophy of technology has recently become a separate discipline, distinct from the philosophy of science or philosophy in general. JAI Press has published an influential series of books on philosophy of technology, and philosophers of technology have been included in major endeavors, such as the Human Genome Project, suggesting recognition of

> The first formal courses outside of engineering schools dealing with technology were developed by departments of history and the philosophy of science.

the importance of philosophy of technology, especially to public policy deliberations.

The NSF through its Science and Technology Studies Program spends about $3 million per year to support research and other activities in the history, philosophy, and social studies of science and technology (Hackett, 2000). NSF's Societal Dimensions of Engineering, Science, and Technology program also supports research on the impacts of technology and engineering.

Management of Technology

A variety of programs at the undergraduate and graduate levels prepare students to assume management responsibilities in technology-based businesses. These programs go by various names, depending on where they are housed in the university. Most are affiliated with an engineering school or a school of management or business. And although the emphasis on engineering-related and management-related topics varies considerably, almost all of these programs blend basic business knowledge with an appreciation for the impact of modern technology on the world of work.

Schools of Education

There are 517 accredited teacher education programs in the United States (NCATE, 2000a). New accreditation standards by the National Council for Accreditation of Teacher Education (NCATE) emphasize that new teachers must have an in-depth knowledge of the subject matter they will teach, the lack of which has been a suspected cause of the poor performance of U.S. students on international assessments of mathematics and science (NCATE, 2000b). Almost one-fifth of U.S. high school teachers who teach science do not have even a minor in science (National Commission on Mathematics and Science Teaching for the 21st Century, 2000). Two hundred twenty schools of education specialize in preparing teachers of science (NCATE, 2000a).

Most of the 80 or so technology teacher education programs in the United States are affiliated with schools of education. NCATE uses program evaluation standards developed by the Council on Technology Teacher Education (CTTE), the professional development arm of the International Technology Education Assocation (ITEA), to review these

> A variety of programs at the undergraduate and graduate levels prepare students to assume management responsibilities in technology-based businesses.

programs for accreditation. The CTTE standards are currently being revised to reflect ITEA's *Standards for Technological Literacy*.

Informal Education

Technological literacy can be improved outside of the formal K-12 or university setting. Most Americans (about 70 percent) are no longer in school, and for them to become more technologically literate, they must have opportunities outside of the school setting, so-called informal educational settings (Figure 4-1).

Museums and science centers, television, radio, newspapers, magazines, and other media comprise the informal education system, which offers citizens of all ages and backgrounds an opportunity to learn about and become engaged in a variety of issues related to technology. Research indicates that formal, school-based education is the primary contributor to a conceptual understanding in the sciences, but informal education also has a measurable impact on the acquisition of science knowledge (Miller, 1998; 2001). Presumably, the same is true for technology.

Museums and Science Centers

The Association of Science-Technology Centers (ASTC), which represents more than 430 institutions around the world, periodically col-

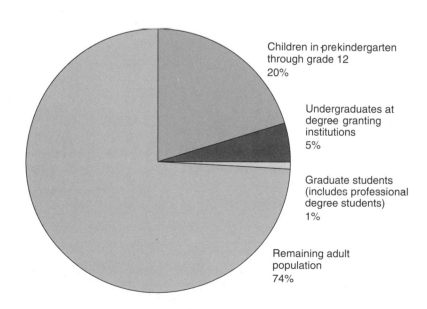

FIGURE 4-1 Educational status of the American population, 2000. Sources: Bairu, 2001; Broughman and Colaciello, 2001; U.S. Census Bureau, 2000.

Children in prekindergarten through grade 12
20%

Undergraduates at degree granting institutions
5%

Graduate students (includes professional degree students)
1%

Remaining adult population
74%

lects information about activities and programs at these facilities. In one survey, 12 percent of the 2,237 exhibits reported by survey participants were considered to be about technology (ASTC, 1997). Technology was the third most popular subject for exhibits, after those in physics and the life sciences. A considerable number of physics exhibits also dealt substantively with technology issues, and many exhibits were grouped in both the physics and technology categories. The greatest number of technology exhibits were related to computers, but a substantial number were focused on communications, energy and power production, and transportation.

Museums and science centers are increasing their educational programs for children and teachers. According to the survey, 83 percent of U.S. ASTC members sponsored teacher education workshops for teachers already working in schools. Museums and science centers also devoted considerable resources to preparing future teachers. More than 40 percent of survey respondents provided museum staff to teach education courses or workshops at local colleges. Thirty-seven percent indicated they were working with universities on education research projects; and nearly 50 percent provided resource kits for training programs for future teachers. A handful of museums produce instructional materials (e.g., San Francisco's Exploratorium).

> Museums and science centers also devoted considerable resources to preparing future teachers.

For years, experts in the science of learning have tried to determine what and how people learn through museum experiences. An estimated 120 million visitors entered science centers and museums in the United States in 2000, suggesting museums play an extremely important role in informal education (ASTC, 2001). However, because visits to museums serve social, entertainment, and educational purposes, and because museum visits are almost always unstructured and of very short duration, it is difficult to quantify how much museum-goers take away from their visits (personal communication, G. Hein, Leslie University, December 17, 2000). Contextual-model based assessments of learning show that museums increase understanding and interest among nearly all visitors (Falk and Dierking, 2000).

Although the primary focus of science and technology centers is on communicating facts and concepts, they can also put issues into a social context and thus engage the public in meaningful debate about the effects of science and technology. A case in point is "Mine Game," an exhibit developed in the early 1990s at Science World in Vancouver, British Columbia (Bradburne, 2000). The exhibit was designed to mirror heated

BOX 4-4 "Engineer It"

The theme of the "Engineer It" exhibit at the Oregon Museum for Science and Industry is "think, build, test, do it again." Funded by NSF and Intel Corporation, the exhibition, which includes a traveling component, is intended to give everyone, especially children, a chance to explore engineering in a practical way. "Engineer It" encourages visitors to use the same steps engineers use to design and build boats, bridges, windmills, and airplanes and then to test their performance in water tanks, shake tables, and wind tunnels. A companion website, <http://www.omsi.org/explore/physics/engineerit/>, provides print and web-based resources for teachers and activities and online games for children.

conflict in the province about the use of natural resources. Museum visitors were challenged to work through competing scenarios of how logging, mining, and environmental protection might coexist.

Exhibits like "Mine Game" are likely to improve technological literacy, especially the dimension of thinking and acting. They engage the public in the messy process of scientific and technological decision making, making concepts such as risk, constraints, and trade-offs of practical value rather than only theoretical importance. Museums and science centers also can contribute to the capabilities dimension of technological literacy, particularly through exhibits that encourage hands-on, problem-solving, and engineering-design activities (Box 4-4).

Television, Radio, Newspapers, and Other Media

Technology as a subject of reporting by print, broadcast, and electronic media is now commonplace. Almost every day, at least one leading story in the local or national news is related to technology. Our fascination with technology is apparent in a ranking of the most important news stories in the twentieth century; almost half involve technology to a substantial degree (Bybee, 2000).

Frequently, the media's focus on technology has a business or consumer slant. The *Washington Post*, for example, has a separate section, <www.Washtech.com>, on its main website devoted to business coverage of technology industries. Like many other newspapers, the *Post*'s print and online coverage of technology often involves developments in computers and other electronic devices. The *New York Times*, *San Jose Mercury News*, *Toronto Star*, and *Seattle Times*, among others, have stand-alone technology sections focused on devices that employ microchips. Even newspapers that do not have stand-alone sections in their print versions often have separate technology sections on their websites (e.g., *Miami Herald*, *San Francisco Chronicle*, *Chicago Tribune*, *USA Today*).

Among television outlets, the Public Broadcasting System (PBS), especially the program "NOVA," has the longest track record of technology-related programming. In the past 20 years, PBS has run dozens of documentaries, special films, and film series on aeronautics and flight, crime, computers, energy, weapons and warfare, and ancient and modern engineering. Many of these programs have companion books, websites, and resources for teachers to use in the classroom. Among cable networks, the Discovery Channel, The History Channel, The Learning Channel, and Think Network have featured technology-related programming. Network television, by and large, has not invested in programming related to technology or, for that matter, science. Notable exceptions are the news magazines, such as 60 Minutes, 60 Minutes II, 48 Hours, Primetime Live, and Dateline, which run occasional in-depth pieces on technology topics.

The Sloan Foundation has funded series of short segments on science and technology topics on Public Radio International and National Public Radio (NPR), as well as segments of "The Osgood File" on CBS radio that relate to technology. According to the Sloan Foundation, at least 20 million listeners tune in to at least one of these broadcasts every week. In 2000, Sloan funded the production of five one-hour radio documentaries on NPR, "The DNA Files," on new developments in genetics.

> Network television, by and large, has not invested in programming related to technology or, for that matter, science.

The Professions

Architects and engineers are well positioned to influence the general level of technological literacy and are already taking steps in this direction. The American Institute of Architects (AIA), for example, compiles a media guide to help editors and reporters cover architecture, interior design, and the building industry. The guide provides contact information for architects around the country who are expert on diverse topics, such as building security, environmental sustainability, and home renovation. Through the American Architectural Foundation, AIA runs a grant program that provides funds to local organizations interested in improving public understanding and appreciation of architecture. The foundation also distributes teacher curriculum guides for grades K-12 that integrate design concepts into science, social studies, art, and other subjects.

A handful of engineering societies have developed and promoted instructional materials for the classroom. One of the most ambitious is the World in Motion series developed for middle schools by the Society for Automotive Engineers (SAE). These eight-week units are focused on problem-solving and design activities. The SAE Foundation supplies activity kits for student experiments, teacher manuals, and instructional videos free of charge to any school that agrees to become partners with a local engineer or company that will provide volunteer support to the classroom.

The Institute of Electrical and Electronics Engineers (IEEE) has been working for the past 3 years to encourage communication and collaboration between practicing engineers and K-12 teachers. The institute recently launched a website, PEERS (Pre-College Engineer/Educator Resource Site; <www.ieee.org/eab/precollege/peers/index/htm>), to facilitate these interactions. In October 2001, IEEE brought together pairs of deans of education and engineering from some 40 universities to consider how technology content might become part of mainstream teacher education and how engineers could become better informed about education theory and practice. IEEE also hosts a comprehensive online resource related to the history of electrical technologies (see Appendix A).

The largest mobilization of engineering talent on behalf of K-12 education occurs during National Engineers Week, held annually during the month of February. A mainstay of the program is the "DiscoverE K-12" program, when 40,000 engineers volunteer in classrooms across the country, interacting with more than five million students and teachers. More than 60 corporations and 75 government, education, engineering and minority organizations supported EWeek 2001.

At least 30 engineering schools or programs in the United States are currently engaged in outreach to the K-12 education community (NAE, unpublished). These initiatives include career days, which bring in schoolchildren to learn about engineering and engineers, summer programs for students and teachers, and visits by university engineers to local classrooms. A few programs, such as the Center for Engineering Educational Outreach at Tufts University, design and disseminate curricula based on engineering principles (see Appendix A).

The health professions, particularly physician groups, are also working to influence the public understanding of technology. Modern

> At least 30 engineering schools or programs in the United States are currently engaged in outreach to the K-12 education community.

medicine has become highly technical, both for practitioners and patients, and many people are poorly equipped to participate in their own care. Recently, the American Medical Association Foundation (2000) launched a campaign to improve communication between doctors and patients, partly by simplifying instructions for and descriptions of medical procedures. Doctor-patient communication about the benefits, risks, and role of technology in health care could easily be made a part of this and similar initiatives.

Contests and Awards

A number of professional societies, businesses, and other organizations sponsor contests and award programs intended to interest students in science, engineering, and technology. The majority of these involve participants in a combination of design, construction, and problem-solving activities. The most well known of contests is the Intel International Science and Engineering Fair, which has been administered by Science Service since 1952. Each year, several million students compete in local, state, and regional fairs around the world. After a lengthy winnowing process, 1,200 finalists vie for cash awards and other prizes in 15 categories, including engineering. The top two contestants receive all-expense-paid trips to attend the Nobel Prize ceremony in Stockholm, Sweden.

> A number of professional societies, businesses, and other organizations sponsor contests to interest students in science, engineering, and technology.

Several contests attempt to attract participants through robotics. The FIRST Robotics Competition, begun by inventor Dean Kamen in the early 1990s, for example, challenges teams of high school students and engineers to design and build a robot that can defeat another robot in some kind of a game. The competition attracts more than 500 teams each year. In 1998, FIRST initiated a contest for middle school children using LEGO building blocks, sensors, motors, and gears.

Real-world problem solving is the focus of the TEAMS (Tests of Engineering Aptitude, Mathematics, and Science) Contest, sponsored by the Junior Engineering Technical Society (JETS). Roughly 1,700 four-to-eight person teams participated last year. Odyssey of the Mind and the Future Problem Solving Contest also emphasize creative problem-solving skills, but students do not participate in hands-on, design-and-build activities.

The National Engineering Design Challenge, sponsored by JETS and several other organizations, encourages the creation of products with practical applications. The finals of this competition, which attracts about 80 teams from around the country, are held in conjunction with National Engineers Week. In the Future City Competition, also part of National Engineers Week, students design a city of the future using SimCity software, build a scale model of part of the city, and propose a solution to a technological problem facing the city.

No one has attempted to assess the impact of these contests on student learning or future career choices, although some programs collect attitudinal or anecdotal information about student participants, their parents, teachers, and coaches. A FIRST survey of participants in the robotics competition found, for example, that 70 percent of the students became more interested in science, and an equal percentage of their parents believe the contest experience was a factor in their children wanting to attend engineering school.

Participation in Technological Decision Making

Several federal agencies have formal mechanisms in place for involving the public in the planning and, sometimes, execution of federally funded projects, some of which have technological aspects. The U.S. Department of Transportation (DOT), for example, requires its grant recipients to provide opportunities for public input on major transportation initiatives. DOT publishes case studies documenting public participation (DOT, 1997a, b, c). Even with these guidelines, however, complex civil works projects can severely test the efforts of local politicians, engineers, and the public at large to work cooperatively (Hughes, 1998).

Applicants for block grant monies from the U.S. Department of Housing and Urban Development (HUD) are required to involve citizens in the planning process for housing, homeless, and community and economic development projects. HUD publishes examples from around the country of best practices related to citizen participation (HUD, 2001). Technology-related issues in HUD-funded projects involve environmental concerns, the design and construction of new buildings, and the revitalization of existing commercial or residential areas.

A number of community organizations in the United States, so-called community-based research groups, initiate, and sometimes participate in and even fund, research projects. This approach is sometimes called "participatory research." Some of these organizations have been active for two decades or more; most are much newer. Because these groups are generally small and independent, it is difficult to gauge the extent of their activities. The Loka Institute, an Amherst-based non-profit, has identified about 75 community-based research organizations around the country, a dozen of which appear to be at least partly concerned with technological issues (Loka Institute, 2001). Many activities by community-based organizations are funded by foundation, university, or local government monies, as well as federal agencies (e.g., CDC, 2001; NIEHS, 2001; USDA, 2001).

International Experience

In some countries, formal mechanisms for involving the public in discussions about the development and use of technology are more common than they are in the United States. Consensus conferences bring together experts and nonexperts to encourage discussions about the scope and implications of technology. Unlike the approach to consensus conferences pioneered by the U.S. National Institutes of Health, in European consensus conferences the conclusions and recommendations are developed by a panel of laypersons, not experts (Van Eijndhoven, 1997).

The Danish Board of Technology (Teknologirådet), which provides technology assessment services to the Danish Parliament, held what was probably the first such consensus conference in the world in 1987, on gene technology in industry and agriculture. To date, the board has sponsored 19 conferences on various topics, including electronic identity cards, educational technology, and the future of private automobiles. A least a dozen other countries, including Japan and South Korea, have attempted to emulate the Danish approach.

Scenario workshops, also pioneered by the Danish Board of Technology, involve the public and other stakeholders—usually business leaders, policy makers, and technical experts—in forward-thinking discussions of the local dimensions of sociotechnical challenges. Scenario workshops are intended to develop solutions to specific problems rather than to explore the use and regulation of technology generally (Andersen and Jaeger, 1999).

The scenario approach was used first in Denmark in the early 1990s to examine the topic of urban ecology. A modified version of the technique, called the European Awareness Scenario Workshop® (EASW), was adapted by the European Commission's (EC) Sustainable Cities and

In some countries, formal mechanisms for involving the public in discussions about the development and use of technology are more common than they are in the United States.

Towns Campaign in 1994. EASW is a tool to help communities respond to the sustainability agenda (Agenda 21), drafted during the Earth Summit in Rio de Janeiro in 1992. EASW scenarios have been developed on four broad themes: the urban environment, regeneration, information and communication, and mobility. In addition, 60 workshops have been held in nine European cities under the auspices of FLEXIMODO, an EC project overseen by a consortium of Dutch, Danish, Italian, and Portuguese organizations (EC, 2000).

Science shops, which originated in the Dutch university system in the mid-1970s, coordinate and sometimes conduct research on social, scientific, and technological issues in response to questions posed by community and public-interest groups as well as by individuals. Public participation in the process is essential, but it is not the overarching purpose. The science-shop approach was developed to engage the academic research community in the solution of societal problems (Utrecht University, 2000).

According to the General Secretariat Dutch Scienceshops, there are 33 science shops at 11 universities in the Netherlands. Each has one or more areas of expertise, such as the environment, physics, chemistry, medicine, or architecture. Science shops or similar organizations are doing work in Denmark, Norway, Germany, Austria, Northern Ireland, England, Canada, South Korea, Malaysia, Israel, and Romania. The EC is currently studying ways to internationalize the science-shop model to increase public access to science (General Secretariat Dutch Scienceshops, 2000).

Another approach, constructive technology assessment (CTA), is designed to include technology users in the technology design process. Rather than focusing on the problems of existing technologies or the potential applications of a technology, CTA focuses on public concerns and desires during the "construction" of a technology. In this respect, CTA is different from other methods of involving lay citizens in technology assessment. The Rathenau Institute (formerly the Netherlands Organisation of Technology Assessment) has been instrumental in the development of the CTA concept. The Dutch government has used the CTA approach to examine the introduction of novel protein foods that could replace meat in the diet. Other countries, notably Denmark, Norway, and Germany, have also used CTA-like processes (Schot and Rip, 1997).

Evidence for Impact

Up to now, very few studies have been done to determine whether the views, concerns, and actions of the nonexpert public actually influence choices about technology. Nor has the effect of such participation on public understanding of science and technology—or on technological literacy—been carefully evaluated. Recently, a small group of mostly European researchers has begun to examine the impact of public participation on decision making. One of the first studies attempted to determine the extent to which consensus conferences influenced the legislative decisions of the Danish Parliament (Joss, 1998). The study involved a mail survey of members of the parliament, follow-up interviews with five of those who responded, and an analysis of parliamentary proceedings and legislation.

The survey showed that 75 percent of members of Parliament had heard of consensus conferences, and half of those had attended at least one. Of those who were familiar with consensus conferences, 13 percent felt that the conferences sometimes led to parliamentary discussions, debates, or initiatives, such as issuance of laws or guidelines. The study documented a number of instances in which consensus conferences were mentioned in parliamentary proceedings or debates. At least one conference, on human genome mapping in 1989, served as the basis for new legislation.

Following a series of Danish scenario workshops in 1992 on urban ecology, the Danish government established a national committee, which is credited with several initiatives encouraging public debate about sustainable housing. But no assessment was done on the long-term effects of the workshops on the communities in which they were held (Andersen and Jaeger, 1999).

An evaluation of the only U.S. participatory consensus conference to date, "Telecommunications and the Future of Democracy," concluded that the conference had "no actual impact" on the substance of telecommunications policy or on the general thinking about the issue among policy makers (Guston, 1998). But the assessment did find that the nonexpert participants in the process learned a good deal about telecommunications technology and about consensus conferences and the role of citizens in public decision making.

Taken together, the available evidence suggests that formal public participation in technological decision making can influence policy

> Very few studies have been done to determine whether the views, concerns, and actions of the nonexpert public actually influence choices about technology.

making, although the effect may be difficult to measure. Public participation does appear to help citizens become more versed in technological matters, at least according to their self-reporting.

Conclusions

The breadth of efforts to boost technological literacy has been impressive. Information to improve the understanding of technology is available in many venues, from kindergarten classrooms to graduate seminars, from news stories in local papers to the exhibit halls of science museums. In terms of promoting the three dimensions of technological literacy, the most extensive efforts have been directed toward the K-12 classroom, for which a cadre of thoughtful technology educators, curriculum developers, and others has produced high-quality instructional materials, textbooks, websites, and other resources. The science standards developed in the early and mid-1990s have provided a framework for integrating science and technology into the classroom, and the newly published ITEA standards for technological literacy could inform teaching and learning about technology for decades to come. For these improvements to be meaningful and lasting, standards, instructional materials, and assessments will have to be coordinated.

Another major impediment to lasting reform is the lack of information about how people, especially students, learn about technology in formal and informal settings. However, interest in the science of learning is burgeoning among educators and policy makers, which is encouraging for the future of technological literacy.

Given the large proportion of citizens who are no longer in school, the informal education system must become a major focus for promoting technological literacy. However, unlike in formal education, where standards, curriculum, and testing govern what is taught, there are no similar pressure points influencing what museums, the media, and others in the informal sector do—or choose to neglect—in their role as educators. An additional concern is the difficulty of determining what people actually learn from exhibits, television programming, or science and technology contests.

The overall situation is discouraging. Many projects have had an impact on student or public understanding of technology but have been of limited duration. And some of the most effective initiatives have reached only a few people. Until a drive for technological literacy is consistently

> For improvements to be meaningful and lasting, standards, instructional materials, and assessments will have to be coordinated.

reinforced in schools and in informal education settings, and until rigorously developed standards, curriculum, and assessments have been developed and put in place, the prospects for sustained improvement are slim.

References

AAAS (American Association for the Advancement of Science). 1989. Science for All Americans. New York: Oxford University Press.

AAAS. 1993. Benchmarks for Science Literacy. New York: Oxford University Press.

American Medical Association Foundation. 2000. Partnership in Health: Improving the Patient-Physician Relationship Through Health Literacy. Available online at: <http://www.ama-assn.org/ama/pub/article/3125-3307.html> (October 5, 2001).

Amram, F. 1989. Poetry as focus for technology, work and values. Pp. 314–324 in Technology Literacy IV: Proceedings of the Fourth National Technological Literacy Conference, edited by D.W. Cheek and L.J. Waks. Bloomington, Ind.: ERIC Clearinghouse for Social Studies/Social Science Education (ED315326).

Andersen, I.-E., and B. Jaeger. 1999. Scenario workshops and consensus conferences: towards more democratic decision-making. Science and Public Policy 26(5): 331–340.

ASTC (Association of Science-Technology Centers). 1997. Yearbook of Science-Center Statistics. Washington, D.C.: ASTC.

ASTC. 2001. ASTC Sourcebook of Science Center Statistics, 2001. Washington, D.C.: ASTC.

Bairu, G. 2001. Public School Student, Staff, and Graduate Counts by State: School Year 1999–2000 (NCES 2001-326r). Washington, D.C.: U.S. Department of Education.

Bradburne, J. 2000. Presentation at Workshop on National and International Efforts that Encourage the Development of Technological Literacy, Committee on Technological Literacy, The National Academies. Washington, D.C., March 16, 2000.

Broughman, S.P., and L.A. Colaciello. 2001. Private School Universe Survey, 1999–2000 (NCES 2001-330). Washington, D.C.: U.S. Department of Education.

BSCS (Biological Sciences Curriculum Study). 1984. Innovations: The Social Consequences of Science and Technology Program. Dubuque, Iowa: Kendall/Hunt Publishing Co.

BSCS. 2000. Science T.R.A.C.S. Dubuque, Iowa: Kendall/Hunt Publishing Co.

Bybee, R. 2000. Achieving technological literacy: A national imperative. The Technology Teacher 60(1): 23–28.

CDC (Centers for Disease Control and Prevention). 2001. Division of Prevention Research and Analytic Methods. Available online at: <http://www.cdc.gov/epo/dpram/dpram.htm> (November 20, 2001).

CORD (Center for Occupational Research and Development). 1984. Principles of Technology. Waco, Texas: CORD.

CORD. 2001. Physics in Context: An Integrated Approach. Waco, Texas: CCI Publishing.

De la Mothe, J.R. 1983. Unity and Diversity in STS Curricula. ED 230–431. Columbus, Ohio: ERIC Clearinghouse on Science, Mathematics, and Environmental Education.

DOT (U.S. Department of Transportation). 1997a. Public Involvement for Transportation Decision-Making—Case Study: South Sacramento, California, Light Rail Transit/La Linea Del Sur. Washington, D.C.: U.S. Government Printing Office.

DOT. 1997b. Public Involvement for Transportation Decision-Making—Case Study: Metroplan (Little Rock, Arkansas) "Pouring Water on Dry Ground." Washington, D.C.: U.S. Government Printing Office.

DOT. 1997c. Public Involvement for Transportation Decision-Making—Case Study: Public Involvement at Oregon Department of Transportation. Washington, D.C.: U.S. Government Printing Office.

EC (European Commission). 2000. Community Research and Development Service, Training and Dissemination Schemes Project. FLEXIMODO. Available online at: <http://www.cordis.lu/tdsp/en/fleximod/00.htm> (November 20, 2001).

Engineering Concepts Curriculum Project. 1971. The Man-Made World. New York: McGraw Hill Publishing.

Fagan, E.R. 1989. Teaching literature: Science/Humanities. Pp. 333–337 in Technology Literacy IV: Proceedings of the Fourth National Technological Literacy Conference, edited by D.W. Cheek and L.J. Waks. Bloomington, Ind.: ERIC Clearinghouse for Social Studies/Social Science Education (ED315326).

Falk, J.H., and L.D. Dierking. 2000. Learning from Museums: Visitor Experiences and the Making of Meaning. Walnut Creek, Calif.: AltaMira Press.

Foltz, F.A. 1988. Origin of an Academic Field: The Science, Technology and Society Paradigm Shift. Unpublished paper in partial fulfillment for M.A. degree. The Pennsylvania State University, University Park, Pa.

General Secretariat Dutch Scienceshops. 2000. National Secretariat Dutch Science Shops. Available online at: <http://www.ssc.unimaas.nl/LSW/indexuk.HTM> (November 20, 2001).

Guston, D.H. 1998. Evaluating the Impact of the First U.S. Citizens' Panel on "Telecommunications and the Future of Democracy." Paper prepared for delivery at the 1998 annual meeting of the American Political Science Association, Boston, September 3-6.

Hackett, E.J. 2000. Trends and opportunities in science and technology studies: A view from the National Science Foundation. Pp. 277–292 in Science, Technology and Society: A Sourcebook on Research and Practice, edited by D.D. Kumar and D.E. Chubin. New York: Kluwer Academic/Plenum Publishers.

Hamm, M., and D. Adams. 1989. An analysis of global problem issues in sixth- and seventh-grade textbooks. Journal of Research in Science Teaching 26(5): 445–452.

Hankins, J.C. 1989. Writing as a bridge between high school science and society: A theoretical perspective. Pp. 344–350 in Technology Literacy IV: Proceedings of the Fourth National Technological Literacy Conference, edited by D.W. Cheek and L.J. Waks. Bloomington, Ind.: ERIC Clearinghouse for Social Studies/Social Science Education (ED315326).

Harkness, J.L., J. Ihde, R. LeClair, and D. Tietge. 1986. Modular Science-Technology-Society. Wausau, Wis.: Modular STS Incorporated.

Harms, N.C., and R.E. Yager. 1981. What Research Says to the Science Teacher. Vol. 3. Washington, D.C.: National Science Teachers Association.

HUD (U.S. Department of Housing and Urban Development). 2001. John J. Gunther Blue Ribbon Practices in Community Development. Topic: Citizen Participation. Available online at: <http://www.hud.gov/ptw/participation.html> (November 13, 2001).

Hughes, T.P. 1998. Coping with complexity: Central Artery/Tunnel. Pp. 197–254 in Rescuing Prometheus. New York: Pantheon Books.

Hughes, T.P. In Press. History of Technology: An Essay for the International Encyclopedia of Social and Behavioral Sciences. Oxford, U.K: Elsevier.

Integrated Mathematics, Science, and Technology. 2001. IMaST home page. Available online at <http://www.ilstu.edu/depts/cemast/imast/imasthome.htm> (November 20, 2001).

Integrating Mathematics, Science, and Technology in the Elementary Schools. 2001. MSTe home page. Available online at <http://www.bnl.gov/scied/mste/mste.html> (June 28, 2001).

ITEA (International Technology Education Association). 2000. Standards for Technological Literacy: Content for the Study of Technology. Reston, Va.: ITEA.

Jasanoff, S., G.E. Markle, J.C. Petersen, and T. Pinch, eds. 1995. Handbook of Science and Technology Studies. Thousand Oaks, Calif.: Sage Publications.

Joss, S. 1998. Danish consensus conferences as a model of participatory technology assessment: an impact study of consensus conferences on Danish Parliament and Danish public debate. Science and Public Policy 25(1): 2–22.

Kumar, D.D., and D.F. Berlin. 1996. A study of STS curriculum implementation in the United States. Science Educator 4(10): 12–19.

Loepp, F., S. Meier, and R. Satchwell. 2000. Integrated program increases test scores. Proceedings of the International Conference of Scholars on Technology Education, edited by G. Graube and W.E. Theuerkauf. Braunschweig, Germany: Technical University Braunschweig.

Loka Institute. 2001. The Community Research Network. Available online at: <http://www.loka.org/crn/index.htm> (November 20, 2001).

Miller, J.D. 1998. The Influence of Science Television and Other Informal Science Education on Civic Scientific Literacy. Paper for a discussion with the staff of NOVA and WGBH, October 23, 1998. Unpublished.

Miller, J.D. 2001. The acquisition and retention of scientific information by American adults. Pp. 93-114 in Free-Choice Science Education: How We Learn Science Outside of School, edited by J.H. Falk. New York: Teachers College Press.

Miller, D.H., and N. Butcher. 1990. Creative environmental dramatic opportunity: An interdisciplinary approach to combine earth science and drama for 8th grade. Pp. 206–209 in Technology Literacy V: Proceedings of the Fifth National Technological Literacy Conference, edited by D.W. Cheek. Bloomington, Ind.: ERIC Clearinghouse for Social Studies/Social Science Education (ED325429).

NAE (National Academy of Engineering). Unpublished. Data collected through an informal survey of engineering schools and engineering programs at U.S. universities, June–August, 2001.

National Commission on Mathematics and Science Teaching for the 21st Century. 2000. Before It's Too Late: A Report to the Nation from the National Commission on Mathematics and Science Teaching for the 21st Century. Available online at: <http://www.ed.gov/americacounts/glenn/report.doc> (November 20, 2001).

National School to Work Office. 2000. Available online at: <http://www.stw.ed.gov> (November 21, 2001).

NCATE (National Council for Accreditation of Teacher Education). 2000a. A List of Professional Accredited Schools, Colleges, and Departments of Education. Washington, D.C.: NCATE.

NCATE. 2000b. NCATE 2000 Unit Standards. Available online at: <http://www.ncate.org/2000/2000stds.pdf> (November 20, 2001).

NCEE (National Commission on Excellence in Education). 1982. A Nation at Risk. Washington, D.C.: U.S. Government Printing Office.

NCES (National Center for Education Statistics). 2000a. Vocational Education in the United States: Towards the Year 2000. Available online at: <http://nces.ed.gov/pubsearch/pubsinfo.asp?pubid=2000029> (November 20, 2001).

NCES. 2000b. IPEDS College Opportunities On-Line. Available online at <www.nces.ed.gov/ipeds/cool> (November 20, 2001).

NIEHS (National Institute of Environmental Health Sciences). 2001. Community-Based Prevention/Intervention Research. Available online at: <http://www.niehs.nih.gov/dert/programs/translat/cbpir/cbpir.htm> (March 5, 2001).

NRC (National Research Council). 1996. National Science Education Standards. Washington, D.C.: National Academy Press.

NSB (National Science Board). 1983. Commission on Precollege Education in Mathematics, Science, and Technology: Educating Americans for the 21st Century. Washington, D.C.: National Science Foundation.

NSB. 2000. Science and Engineering Indicators 2000—Volume 1. National Science Board. Arlington, Va.: National Science Foundation.

NSSB (National Skill Standards Board). 2000. The NSSB: A Brief Description. Available online at: <http://www.nssb.org/> (November 20, 2001).

NSTA (National Science Teachers Association). 1982. Science-Technology-Society: Science Education for the 1980s. Washington, D.C.: NSTA.

Piel, E.J. 1981. Interaction of science, technology and society in secondary schools. Pp. 94–112 in What Research Says to the Science Teacher, Vol. 3, edited by N.C. Harms and R.E. Yager. Washington, D.C.: National Science Teachers Association.

Schot, J., and A. Rip. 1997. The past and future of constructive technology assessment. Technological Forecasting and Social Change 54: 251–68.

SHOT (Society for the History of Technology). 2000. Available online at: <http://www.press.jhu.edu/associations/shot/index.htm> (November 20, 2001).

Tangum, M. 1989. Writing to learn: An NSF summer experience. Pp. 362–370 in Technology Literacy IV: Proceedings of the Fourth National Technological Literacy Conference, edited by D.W. Cheek and L.J. Waks. Bloomington, Ind.: ERIC Clearinghouse for Social Studies/Social Science Education (ED315326).

Todd, R., and P. Hutchinson. 2000. The transfer of design and technology to the United States: A case study. Pp. 215–223 in Design and Technology International Millennium Conference 2000, edited by R. Kimbell. Wellesborne, England: The Design and Technology Association.

U.S. Census Bureau. 2000. Population Estimates Program, Population Division, Washington, D.C. Available online at: <http://www.census.gov/population/www/index.html> (June 28, 2001).

USDA (U.S. Department of Agriculture). 2001. USDA Forest Service. Urban and Community Forest Ecosystem Research. Urban Forest Research Units. Available online at: <http://svinet2.fs.fed.us/ne/syracuse/otherfs.html> (November 13, 2001).

Utrecht University. 2000. Introduction, Utrecht Scienceshops (English translation). Available online at: <http://www.uu.nl/cws/english/homepage.html> (November 20, 2001).

Van Eijndhoven, J.C.M. 1997. Technology assessment: Product or process? Technological Forecasting and Social Change 54: 269–286.

Yager, R.E. 1996. History of science/technology/society as reform in the United States. Pp. 3–15 in Science/Technology/Society as Reform in Science Education, edited by R.E. Yager. Albany: State University of New York Press.

5

Recommendations

Based on direct and indirect evidence from a variety of sources, as well as committee members' experiences and expert judgment, the committee concluded that it is in the interest of all Americans to understand more about technology. The conclusion is based on an exploration of technology's role in society and our relationship to it; an analysis of how current social, political, and educational environments affect both the idea and the practical expression of technological literacy; an estimation of the benefits—to individuals and society at large—of greater technological literacy; and a sampling of initiatives that may provide a foundation for a more serious and sustained campaign for technological literacy. The logical question, then, is, what comes next? What steps should be taken, and by whom, to make a campaign for technological literacy a reality? The ultimate goal of the campaign must be to increase the number of people who are knowledgeable, thoughtful, and capable with respect to technology (Figure 5-1).

The Committee on Technological Literacy decided to focus its recommendations on four areas: (1) formal and informal education; (2) research; (3) decision making; and (4) educational innovation. While more categories are possible, the committee believes this set provides an appropriate, balanced, and feasible agenda for enhancing technological literacy in the United States. The categories are addressed roughly in order of priority. Readers should note, however, that the recommendations overlap and support each other, so no category can be ignored. For instance, the availability of better data about technological literacy and how people learn about technology will inform efforts in the education sector. Initiatives to improve technological decision making, which would

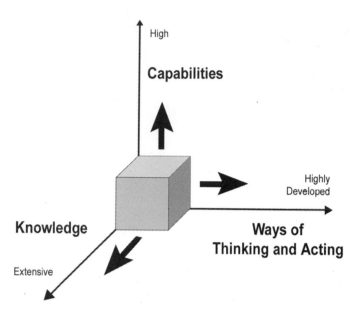

FIGURE 5-1 The dimensions of technological literacy, showing desired growth in the "space" occupied by most Americans.

increase public awareness of the value of informed debate about technology, should also increase support for research and educational reforms.

Strengthening the Presence of Technology in Formal and Informal Education

The U.S. education system has many components that are closely interrelated. Creating lasting change in this complex system requires a strategy that targets several components simultaneously over a sustained period of time. Four key points in the system are curricula, instructional materials, student testing, and standards. Currently, few curricula or instructional materials at the K-12 or undergraduate level integrate nontechnology subjects with technology-related content. Short of the widespread adoption of dedicated courses in technology—an unlikely scenario, in the committee's view—the inclusion of technology subject matter in other academic areas is one of the surest ways of increasing the visibility of technology in U.S. schools. To date, the most attention has been paid to integrating technology with science and mathematics. The committee urges that these initiatives be continued, and, in addition, attempts should be made to include technology content in other subjects, such as social studies, civics, history, geography, art, language arts, and even literature.

There are virtually no tests at the state, national, or international level designed to measure what K-12 students and undergraduates know about technology. As curricula and instructional materials that incorporate technology content are developed, questions about technology are likely to be integrated into student assessments. In addition, targeted efforts to redesign these tests to include technology-related items could significantly accelerate the integration of technological content into curricula.

Although national standards in a variety of subject areas, such as science, mathematics, history, and language arts, stress connections to technology, for the most part these standards are not reflected in the curricula, instructional materials, and assessments for those subjects. State curriculum frameworks for most school subjects do not make connections to technology content.

Recommendation 1 Federal and state agencies that help set education policy should encourage the integration of technology content into K-12 standards, curricula, instructional materials, and student assessments in nontechnology subject areas.

At the federal level, the National Science Foundation (NSF) and the Department of Education (DoEd) can do this in a number of ways, including, when appropriate, making integration a requirement for providing funding for the development of curriculum and instructional materials. The technically oriented federal agencies (e.g., National Aeronautics and Space Administration, the Departments of Agriculture, Commerce, Defense, and Energy, National Institutes of Health, Food and Drug Administration, Occupational Safety and Health Administration) can support integration by developing background materials for teachers of science, history, social studies, civics, the arts, and language arts keyed to national standards and benchmarks in those subjects.

At the state level, science and technology advisors and advisory councils can use their influence with governors, state legislatures, and industry to encourage the inclusion of technology content in nontechnology subjects, not only in the general K-12 curriculum but also in school-to-work and technician-preparation programs. State boards of education can provide incentives for publishers to modify next-generation science, history, social studies, civics, and language arts textbooks to include technology content, for example by incorporating technological themes into state educational standards or by modifying the criteria for school textbooks to include a requirement that the texts contain substantial technology content. Science and history tests that are part of the National Assessment of Educational Progress and future iterations of the Third International Mathematics and Science Survey could be modified to include technology-related items.

Science and technology are so closely connected in the modern world that it is hard to think about them as separate entities. This interconnectedness may explain the confusion in the minds of students, teachers, and the public at large about how science and technology are related. Both have played fundamental roles in our history and culture. In the vast majority of U.S. classrooms, however, technology is not treated as a partner to science or recognized as a major influence on society. Some science classes touch on design, problem solving, and other facets of technological thinking, but teachers and instructional materials rarely explore these concepts. Even fewer nonscience curricula and instructional materials touch on technology.

Recommendation 2 The states should better align their K-12 standards, curriculum frameworks, and student assessment in the sciences, mathematics, history, social studies, civics, the arts, and language arts with national educational standards that stress the connections between these subjects and technology. NSF- and DoEd-funded instructional materials and informal-education initiatives should also stress these connections.

State boards of education in the United States should explicitly link K-12 content in the sciences, mathematics, history, social studies, civics, the arts, and language arts with technology content in their standards, curriculum frameworks, and student assessments in ways suggested by the appropriate national standards. (For example, in science, boards of education might refer to *Benchmarks for Science Literacy*, the *National Science Education Standards*, and the *Standards for Technological Literacy: Content for the Study of Technology*. In mathematics, boards could refer to *Principles and Standards for School Mathematics*.) State science and technology advisors and advisory councils should use their influence with governors, state legislatures, industry, and community colleges to support and facilitate this process.

All new instructional materials developed with funding from NSF, DoEd, or other federal agencies should have a much more sophisticated and expanded presentation of technological concepts and themes, and these should be closely articulated with the materials' core content in the sciences or other subjects.

In a parallel action, federally funded projects in informal education, particularly those supported by the NSF, should be required to make explicit the relationship between technology and the main academic subject focus of the initiative, as spelled out in the appropriate national standards.

A better understanding of the distinctions between science and technology as well as their interdependencies would enable teachers to focus their efforts on technological design issues in the classroom, which could lead to more discussion of attitudes and assumptions about technology. Teachers and students could then focus on related questions about the risks and benefits of introducing new technologies, ethical issues, issues of evidence, and so on.

Recommendation 3 NSF, DoEd, state boards of education, and others involved in K-12 science education should introduce, where appropriate, the word "technology" into the titles and contents of science standards, curricula, and instructional materials.

This seemingly trivial change in language could have a profound effect on students' and the public's awareness of technology. This recommendation *is not a recommendation for new courses.* The change would be appropriate in many cases where the word "science" appears in isolation. The addition of the word "technology" would provide a more accurate description of the content of some curricula and would put technology issues on an equal footing, at least linguistically, with science issues.

Another crucial component in the U.S. educational system is teacher education. Indeed, the success of changes in curricula, instructional materials, and assessments will depend largely on the ability of teachers to implement those changes. Lasting improvements will require both the creation of new teaching and assessment tools as well as the appropriate preparation of teachers to use those tools effectively.

Recommendation 4 NSF, DoEd, and teacher education accrediting bodies should provide incentives for institutions of higher education to transform the preparation of all teachers to better equip them to teach about technology throughout the curriculum.

In general, teachers of technology must approach the subject from an engineering perspective rather than an industrial arts perspective. These teachers must be fully conversant with the International Technology Education Association's *Standards for Technological Literacy* and familiar with the materials and techniques for teaching to those standards. Technology teachers with a good understanding of science and the interactions between technology, science, and society will be well prepared to work with other teachers to integrate technology with other subjects.

Teachers of science should have a solid education in technology and engineering design to ensure that they are prepared to use new materials that will become available that include technology-related examples and activities. Teachers of history and social studies should be required to become knowledgeable about how science and technology influence history and society.

Elementary school teachers should, at the very least, be scientifically and technologically literate. Universities can provide appropriate courses or make provisions for teachers to meet this requirement by examination. The content of the American Assocation for the Advancement of Science's (AAAS) *Science for All Americans* could be used as a minimum standard; the publications listed in AAAS's *Resources for Science Literacy* (Appendix A) can provide some of the necessary information.

Teachers at all levels should be able to conduct design projects and use design-oriented teaching strategies to encourage learning.

Developing a Research Base

Efforts to improve technological literacy in the United States have been hampered by a weak research base. The lack of reliable, longitudinal information about what people know and believe about technology, for example, has made it difficult for curriculum developers to design strategies for addressing gaps in what students know, correcting misconceptions, and building on existing understandings. Further, because we have not been able to measure changes in public understanding, policy makers have been hard pressed to know how to enhance technological literacy.

Very little research has been done on the cognitive steps involved in constructing new knowledge about technology. This information would benefit developers of instructional materials and curricula, as well as teachers trying to plan classroom strategies and designers of initiatives in informal education. Developing a research base for technological literacy will require creating cadres of competent researchers, developing and periodically revising a research agenda, allocating funding for research projects, and incorporating research findings in teaching materials and techniques.

Recommendation 5 NSF should support the development of assessment tools that can be used to monitor the state of technological literacy among students and the public in the United States.

> NSF, which has already invested considerable effort in determining the public understanding of, and attitudes toward, science and technology, should take the lead in supporting assessment research. A first step would be to evaluate methods currently used to measure knowledge and understanding in other subject areas to determine if they could be used to gauge technological literacy. Researchers would have to take into account the special challenges associated with assessing technological understanding, including the different meanings people attribute to the word "technology" and the real, sometimes confusing connections between science and technology. Researchers should also consider how much an assessment of technological literacy should rely on knowledge and capabilities spelled out in formal content standards (e.g., the standards created by the International Technology Education Association, National Research Council, and American Association for the Advancement of Science).

Recommendation 6 NSF and DoEd should fund research on how people learn about technology, and the results should be applied in formal and informal education settings.

This research would focus on the relationship between scientific knowledge and technological knowledge; the roles of procedural and conceptual knowledge in enhancing technological understanding; the nature and process of technological problem solving; and the application of findings in cognitive science to technological learning. The work being done by the American Association for the Advancement of Science to develop a research agenda for technology education should be continued and expanded.

The results of this research must be translated into practical strategies for enhancing learning and teaching in the classroom and in informal settings, such as museums, science and technology centers, and through materials in print, online, and in the broadcast media.

Enhancing Informed Decision Making

In a modern nation like the United States, a substantial number of decisions have a technological component. Outside the formal school setting, one of the best ways to become educated about technology is to engage in discussions of the pros and cons, risks and benefits, knowns and unknowns of a particular technology or technological choice. Engagement in decision making is likely to have a direct, positive effect on the nonexpert participants, and involving the nonexpert public in deliberations about technological developments as they are taking shape, rather than after the fact, may actually shorten the time and reduce the resources required to bring new technologies into service. Equally important, public participation may also result in design changes that better reflect the needs and desires of society.

Recommendation 7 Industry, federal agencies responsible for carrying out infrastructure projects, and science and technology museums should provide more opportunities for the nontechnical public to become involved in discussions about technological developments.

The technical community—especially engineers and scientists in industry—is largely responsible for the amount and quality of communication and outreach to the public on technological issues. Industry should err on the side of encouraging greater public engagement, even if it may not always be clear what types of technological development merit public input. In the federal arena, some agencies already require recipients of funding to engage communities likely to be affected by planned infrastructure projects. These efforts should be expanded. In general, efforts to enhance public involvement in technological decision making in the United States could benefit from the experiences of other nations, particularly Denmark and Holland.

The informal education sector, especially museums and science and technology centers, is well positioned to prepare the nontechnical public to grapple with the complexities of decision making in the technological realm. These institutions and the government agencies, companies, and foundations that support them could do much more to encourage public discussion and debate about the direction and nature of technological development at both the local and national level.

Informed decision making is important for all citizens of a democracy and is vital for leaders in government and industry whose decisions influence the health and welfare of the nation. State and federal legislators, who set policy and allocate resources, largely determine the national agenda in education, national security, health care, and many other areas. Industry shapes the consumer culture and drives economic growth and productivity through investments in research, product development, and marketing.

Government and industry both face a daunting array of issues with substantial technological components, from the creation and regulation of genetically modified organisms to the future of the Internet and e-commerce. The committee believes there is a great unmet need in both sectors for information and education that would contribute to more informed decision making about technological matters.

Recommendation 8 Federal and state government agencies with a role in guiding or supporting the nation's scientific and technological enterprise, and private foundations concerned about good governance, should support executive education programs intended to increase the technological literacy of government and industry leaders.

Executive education programs could include courses, lasting from several days to several weeks, designed for leaders and decision makers (and key staff) in Congress, state and local governments, and industry. The courses might use case studies to deal with current and anticipated technological problems and choices. These courses could be offered in many locations throughout the country, at major research universities, community colleges, law schools, business schools, schools of management, colleges of engineering, and other institutions. The courses would be taught by experts in technology, science, history of science and technology, and technological literacy.

The engineering community, which is directly involved in the creation of technology, is uniquely equipped to promote technological literacy. An engineering-led effort to increase technological literacy could have significant, long-term pay-offs, not only for decision makers in government but also for the public at large.

Recommendation 9 U.S. engineering societies should underwrite the costs of establishing government- and media-fellow programs with the goal of creating a cadre of policy experts and journalists with a background in engineering.

These programs could be small to begin with, but should be expanded over time to include a larger number of fellows from the ranks of master's, doctoral, and postdoctoral level engineers. Government fellowship programs could include workshops and internships in Congress and statehouses around the country. Because few national or state legislators are engineers, a technologically savvy staff could be very helpful. Graduates of the program might become permanent government employees or might return to engineering practice or education but would continue to serve as consultants to state and local legislators on technological issues.

The training for media fellows should include workshops, followed by internships at cooperating newspapers, magazines, or television or radio stations. Graduates of the program might become professional journalists or might return to engineering, but would continue to serve as consultants to the media. Better media coverage of technological issues would help inform citizens, who would then be better equipped to make decisions in their own lives.

Rewarding Teaching Excellence and Educational Innovation

One of the biggest obstacles to enhancing technological literacy in the United States is the limited amount of high-quality instructional materials and curricula available. Although some good materials and effective curricula and programs have been developed, the developers often do not have sufficient funding, time, or expertise to disseminate their work to a broad audience. Some teachers, education researchers, and curriculum developers have created interesting and effective approaches to engaging students in technology and design activities, but most of them are known only in the school or school system where they originated.

Recommendation 10 NSF, in collaboration with industry partners, should provide funding for awards for innovative, effective approaches to improving the technological literacy of students or the public at large.

A key criterion for the awards should be that the innovation be scalable (i.e., it can be replicated on a large scale). The awards would provide financial and logistical support for disseminating the innovation widely across the United States. The National Academy of Engineering's Gordon Prize, which is awarded for innovations in engineering education, could be a model for developing an award program.

For almost 20 years, outstanding teachers in science and mathematics from around the United States have been recognized annually for their contributions to student learning through the Presidential Awards for Excellence in Math and Science Teaching. Awardees receive a $7,500 educational grant for their schools, a presidential citation, and a trip to Washington, D.C., for a series of events honoring their achievements. The program not only increases the visibility of the work of high-caliber teachers, it also draws public attention to and helps build support for excellence in science and math education. No similar award exists for technology education.

Recommendation 11 The White House should add a Presidential Award for Excellence in Technology Teaching to those that it currently offers for mathematics and science teaching.

The NSF, which administers the Presidential Awards for Excellence in Mathematics and Science Teaching for the White House, should consult with the International Technology Education Association (ITEA), which already has several long-standing award programs for technology teachers who are members of the organization. Those eligible for the new award could include not only teachers with degrees in technology education, but also teachers with backgrounds in science, math, and other subjects.

A Final Word

The purpose of this report is to inform the public—and especially people in a position to affect policy—of the urgent need for technological literacy. The report and its recommendations provide only a starting point. The case for technological literacy must be made consistently, on an ongoing basis, in light of the technological developments of the time. As Americans gradually become more sophisticated with regard to technological issues, they will be more willing to support measures in the schools and in the informal education arena to raise the level of technological literacy of the next generation. In time, leaders in government, academia, and business will also recognize the value of widespread technological literacy to their own and the nation's welfare. The journey promises to be slow and challenging but unquestionably worth the effort.

APPENDIX A
Toolkit for
Technological Literacy

This appendix is a compilation of resources—a toolkit— intended to assist readers who want to know more about technology and technological literacy. The toolkit is a sampling rather than a comprehensive listing. Most of these sources of information will be of interest to general audiences; some may be of more interest to specific groups. Educators, for example, may find the "Resources for the K-12 Classroom" particularly useful. An expanded and updated version of the toolkit is available on the National Academy of Engineering website that accompanies this report: <www.nae.edu/techlit>.

The Committee on Technological Literacy and project staff have reviewed these entries for relevance and accuracy. However, inclusion on this list does not represent an endorsement by either the committee or the National Academies or a judgment of the quality of a particular organization or resource.

Nature and History of Technology

Autonomous Technology: Technics-out-of-Control as a Theme in Political Thought
Langdon Winner, Massachusetts Institute of Technology Press, 1977.

This book explores the relationship between technology and political theory throughout history. Winner stresses the interactions between technology and conceptions of human nature and social and political institutions.

Beyond Engineering: How Society Shapes Technology
Robert Pool, Oxford University Press, 1997.

This book, part of the Sloan Foundation Technology Book Series, presents the fascinating, often complex ways machines and society interact. Pool demonstrates that technology is shaped not only by engineering, but also by cultural values, economics, management, and history.

Buildings, Bridges, and Tunnels
<www.discovery.com/stories/technology/buildings/buildings.html>

This website explores how tall buildings have evolved through time, tours grand bridges around the world, and explains tunnel technologies. This is a companion site to a three-part series on the Discovery Channel celebrating the advances in engineering design and technology.

Designing Engineers
Louis L. Bucciarelli, MIT Press, 1996.

X-ray inspection systems at airports, photoprint machines, and a residential energy system all illustrate how society influences engineering design. Through case studies, readers are shown how business and management issues, as well as engineering design, influence the conceptualization and production of technologies.

The Design of Everyday Things
Donald A. Norman, Currency/Doubleday, 1990.

This collection of examples of good and bad design includes some simple rules for designers and prompts readers to think about how they interact with their surroundings.

Does Technology Drive History?: The Dilemma of Technological Determinism
Edited by Merritt Roe Smith and Leo Marx, MIT Press, 1994.

The essays in this collection focus on how society is shaped by technology. Experts in various disciplines argue that technologies are social products and therefore subject to social or democratic controls.

Dream Reaper: The Story of an Old-Fashioned Inventor in the High-Tech, High-Stakes World of Modern Agriculture
Craig Canine, Alfred A. Knopf, 1995.

In the past 150 years, agricultural technology has changed dramatically as the population has moved from farms into cities. The author describes those changes through the struggle of two cousins from Kansas who developed and marketed a new type of grain reaper.

Engineering and the Mind's Eye
Eugene S. Ferguson, MIT Press, 1994.

Focusing on design and visualization, Ferguson argues that good engineering relies as much on intuition and imagination as on models and calculations. The author presents the story of engineering as a profession and argues that engineering education must prepare engineers for working on projects in the real world, as opposed to models and theories.

The Existential Pleasures of Engineering (Second Edition)
Samuel Florman, St. Martin's Press, 1995.

This book explores the thoughts and feelings of engineers about their profession and their work. Florman also discusses some philosophies of technology.

The Great Idea Finder
<www.ideafinder.com>

The Great Idea Finder (TGIF) website highlights historic and cutting-edge inventions, profiles inventors, and provides resources for learning about technology and innovation.

Greatest Achievements of the 20th Century
<www.greatachievements.org/greatachievements>

From electricity and safe drinking water to airplanes and computers, engineering reshaped society in the twentieth century. This website provides pictures and background material on 20 of the most important engineering achievements of the last hundred years.

High Tech, High Touch: Technology and Our Search for Meaning
John Naisbitt, Nana Naisbitt, and Douglas Philips, Broadway Books, 1999.

This book presents information on technological issues and includes interviews with doctors, scientists, military leaders, and clergy, who believe that technology is accelerating the pace of activity and feeding the yearning for more emotionally satisfying lives.

How Stuff Works
<www.howstuffworks.com>

This website provides information about how everything from computers to coffeemakers works. It includes a question of the day archive, feature articles that change regularly, and a HowStuffWorks Express site for kids.

The Intellectual Appropriation of Technology: Discourses on Modernity, 1900–1939
Edited by Mikael Hård and Andrew Jamison, MIT Press, 1998.

The essays in this collection suggest that current debates about technology have been shaped by the social and academic responses to techonological developments from 1900–1940. The authors focus on how attitudes about technology are shaped by national and cultural traditions.

The Invention That Changed the World: How a Small Group of Radar Pioneers Won the Second World War and Launched a Technological Revolution
Robert Buderi, Simon & Schuster, 1996.

Buderi recounts the rapid development of radio detection and ranging (RADAR) during World War II and the subsequent scientific and technological advances it inspired. This story includes technical details, as well as descriptions of the personalities, rivalries, and broader context that influenced the development of this seminal technology.

Longitude: The True Story of a Lone Genius Who Solved the Greatest Scientific Problem of His Time
Dava Sobel, Walker and Company, 1998.

This is the remarkable story of a clock maker who invented the chronometer, which revolutionized navigation at sea.

More Work for Mother: The Ironies of Household Technology from the Open Hearth to the Microwave
Ruth Schwartz Cowan, Basic Books, 1983.

As people moved away from traditional farming, many labor-saving devices were developed to help with chores that had been done by men or children. Cowan argues that the roles of family members in household maintenance have changed much more slowly than the technology, which ironically has increased the responsibility of women.

Paths of Innovation: Technological Change in 20th Century America
David C. Mowery and Nathan Rosenberg, Cambridge University Press, 1998.

The internal combustion engine, electricity, and chemistry are a few of the case studies in this book on innovation in America in the twentieth century. The authors also identify general patterns of techonological development and economic growth.

The Religion of Technology: The Divinity of Man and the Spirit of Invention
David F. Noble, A.A. Knopf, 1997.

Noble's thesis is that science and religion were closely linked for most of the 2000 years of Western history. When science became a quest for knowledge separate from its religious underpinnings, he argues, technical progress took off in a different direction, sometimes leading to terrible events like Hiroshima and Chernobyl.

Rescuing Prometheus: Four Monumental Projects That Changed the Modern World
Thomas P. Hughes, Pantheon Books, 1998.

Hughes tells the story of how four large-scale techonological projects undertaken since World War II have contributed to new methods of management and engineering. He argues that innovation is now the product of interacting systems of technology rather than of an inventor working alone.

Sightseer's Guide to Engineering
<www.engineeringsights.org>

This online travel guide includes links to websites for manufacturing facilities, roller coasters, ski lifts, museums, lighthouses, and engineering marvels like the Golden Gate Bridge and Hoover Dam. The site is sponsored by the National Society of Professional Engineers and National Engineers Week.

The Soul of a New Machine
Tracy Kidder, Modern Library, 1997.

This Pulitizer Prize winning book follows a group of young

engineers at Data General who built a new minicomputer in just one year. Their handling of the difficult and complex obstacles to achieve this goal set a standard of highly motivated, hard-working professionals in the computer industry.

Technology and Culture

This international quarterly journal published by the Society for the History of Technology includes articles on the history of technology and its relationship to politics, economics, labor, business, the environment, public policy, science, and the arts. Details, including subscription information, are available at <shot.jhu.edu/tc.html>.

Technology and the Future (Eighth Edition)
Edited by Albert H. Teich., Bedford/St. Martin's Press, 2000.

The essays in this collection were written by scholars of technology and society with a variety of opinions about the future relationship between them. The essays focus on theories, limits, and risks of technology and impacts on medicine, labor, politics and policy, society, gender roles, and the family.

Technological Literacy
Edited by Michael J. Dryenfurth and Michael R. Kozak, Council on Technology Teacher Education, MacMillan/McGraw-Hill, 1991.

This collection of essays covers the context for technological literacy, provides different perspectives on the concept, and suggests practical implications for technology educators.

Technopoly: The Surrender of Culture to Technology
Neil Postman, Vintage Books, 1993.

In this book, Postman argues that the United States has become the world's first technopoly—a culture that not only uses technology, but is also shaped by it.

To Engineer Is Human: The Role of Failure in Successful Design
Henry A Petroski, Vintage Books, 1993.

Petroski uses several examples to demonstrate that engineering successes are often the results of a long succession of sometimes spectacular, but forgotten, failures.

The Unbound Prometheus: Technological Change and Industrial Development in Western Europe from 1750 to the Present
David S. Landes, Cambridge University Press, 1969.
This classic book presents basic economic issues and techonological change that have had the greatest impact on society since 1750.

Virtual Center for Science and Technology
<echo.gmu.edu/center>
Exploring and Collecting History Online (ECHO) Virtual Center for Science and Technology is an annotated catalogue of Internet sites on the history of science, technology, and medicine. This resource includes links from the original WWW Virtual Library.

Why Things Bite Back: Technology and the Revenge of Unintended Consequences
Edward Tenner, Alfred A. Knopf, 1996.
Using examples from sports, medicine, environmental control, and the computerized office, Tenner describes how new technologies can have unexpected results, such as unforeseen problems and unforeseen benefits.

Resources for the K-12 Classroom

Building Big
<www.pbs.org/wgbh/buildingbig/index.html>
BUILDING BIG™ explores the history of some of the greatest feats of engineering in the world and the ingenuity of the engineers, architects, and builders who designed and built them. This is a companion site to a five-part PBS series.

The Children Designing & Engineering Project
The College of New Jersey; 103 AR, P.O. Box 7718, Ewing, NJ 08628-0718; Phone: 609-771-3331; Email: hutchinp@tcnj.edu.
The Children Designing & Engineering Project is a collaboration of the College of New Jersey's Department of Technological Studies, the New Jersey Chamber of Commerce, and the Institute of Electrical and Electronics Engineers. The project has developed instructional materials for the K-5 age group using a thematic design-and-technology approach. The hands-on, inquiry-based units emphasize the relationship between

science, math, technology, and the business world. They range between four and six weeks in length and take approximately 15-20 hours to complete. Details available at: <http://www.tcnj.edu/~cde/home.html>.

The City Technology Project

City College of New York; 140ᵗʰ St. & Convent Ave.; Room T-233; New York, NY 10031. Phone: 212-650-8389 Email: citytechnology@ccny.cuny.edu.

The City Technology Project is a collaboration of elementary classroom teachers, the City College Schools of Education and Engineering, the Center for Children and Technology and the Institute of Electrical and Electronics Engineers. The project has developed materials for teachers to support the teaching of technology in the elementary grades. These materials draw upon everyday artifacts and systems as the source of materials for analysis and design. Five volumes in the *Stuff that Works!* series are available from Heinemann (Portsmouth, NH): *Mechanisms & Other Systems*; *Packaging & Other Structures*; *Mapping*; *Designed Environments: Places, Practices and Plans*; and *Signs, Symbols & Codes*. The project is currently organizing a professional development plan to support the use of these materials through hands-on workshops and Internet-based forums.

DESIGN

Harvard-Smithsonian Center for Astrophysics; Science Education Department, MS-71, 60 Garden Street, Cambridge, MA 02138; Phone: 617-496-4796; Email: hcoyle@cfa.harvard.edu

Doable engineering science investigations geared for nonscience students (DESIGN) are design-based activity modules for use in physical science and technology courses in grades 5 through 9. The engineering projects include: batteries, bridges, electromagnets, gravity cars, solar houses, and windmills. Students make prototypes of specific designs and are then challenged to improve them in some way, such as by increasing their speed while working within constraints, such as size or budget. DESIGN II is a one-year physical science and technology course for middle schools, based on the engineering projects developed and tested through the DESIGN project. Details are available at: <cfa-www.harvard.edu/cfa/sed/projects/designsinfo.html>.

EngineerGirl

<www.engineergirl.org>

This site for girls about engineers and engineering careers features a Gallery of Women Engineers, an Ask an Engineer option, a career quiz, and an increasing number of engineering links. A companion website, Celebration of Women in Engineering <www.nae.edu/cwe>, provides additional project plans and resources for parents, teachers, and other mentors.

Integrated Mathematics, Science, and Technology

Center for Mathematics, Science, and Technology; Illinois State University, Campus Box 5960, Normal, IL 61790-5000; Phone: 309-438-3089; Email: cemast@ilstu.edu

The Integrated Mathematics, Science, and Technology (IMaST) program provides an integrated curriculum for grades 6 through 8 that promotes hands-on learning for students and teamwork among teachers from different disciplines. Teams of mathematics, science, and technology specialists, in collaboration with experts in other fields, researched and created this curriculum that meets national standards. Details are available at: <www.ilstu.edu/depts/cemast/imast/imasthome.htm>.

Integrating Technology Education Across the Curriculum

Many NSF-funded curricula and teacher-developed classroom activities are catalogued in this annotated list of technology education resources, programs, and publications. The list is available through the International Technology Education Association and can be accessed through its website at: <www.iteawww.org>.

Learning by Design

The EduTech Institute; Georgia Institute of Technology, 801 Atlantic Drive, Atlanta, GA 30332; Phone: 404-894-3807; Email: mamie@cc.gatech.edu

In the Learning by Design approach to math and science, students learn through collaborative design activities and reflection on their experiences. The bases for these project-based curriculum units for middle school classrooms are complex, real-world engineering and design problems. Researchers at Georgia Tech's EduTech Institute, working with teachers from Atlanta-area school systems, developed units including: Vehicles in Motion, Work and Energy, Machines That Help, Managing

Erosion, Tunneling, and Changing Coastlines. Details are available at: <www.cc.gatech.edu/edutech/projects/lbdview.html>.

Manufacturing Is Cool!

<www.manufacturingiscool.com/>

Information on colleges, engineering camps for students, facility tours, scholarships, and classroom resources are available on this site, which focuses on careers and opportunities in manufacturing.

Middle School Science and Technology

BSCS; 5415 Mark Dabling Boulevard, Colorado Springs, CO 80918-3842; Phone: 719-531-5550; Email: info@bscs.org

The Biological Sciences Curriculum Study (BSCS) Middle School Science and Technology curriculum materials are designed to incorporate technology, including principles of design, cost-and-benefit and systems analysis, and complexity into technological problems. Details may be found at: <www.bscs.org>.

NASA Education Programs

<http://ehb2.gsfc.nasa.gov/edcats/2000/nep/programs/index.html>

Like several other organizations and government agencies, the National Aeronautics and Space Administration (NASA) supports education programs relating to technology. This website is a comprehensive list of NASA's education programs.

Resources for Science Literacy: Professional Development

American Association for the Advancement of Science, Oxford University Press, 1997.

This resource book includes an extensive list of science trade books on the nature of technology and the designed world. The book comes with a CD-ROM that contains additional information and book reviews. It can be ordered through AAAS's Project 2061 website at: <www.project2061.org>.

SMETE Open Federation

SMETE Open Federation Headquarters; 3115 Etcheverry Hall, University of California at Berkeley; Berkeley, CA 94720-1750; Phone: 510-643-1818; Website: <www.smete.org>

SMETE.ORG is developing a digital library to provide students, teachers, other education professionals, and lifelong learners access to a comprehensive collection of science, mathematics, engineering and technology (SMET) education content online.

The Technology Teacher Magazine

Published eight times a year, this journal is for technology education professionals from elementary school teachers to middle school, junior high, and high school classroom teachers, as well as educators of teachers. Articles cover many issues, including technology learning activities, new programs, and reports of current trends in technology education. Subscription information is available online at: <www.iteawww.org/F1.html>.

TIES Magazine

The online Magazine of Design & Technology Education (TIES) provides stories and ideas for integrating math, science, and technology in middle, junior, and senior high school curricula. Articles emphasize design and problem solving as instructional techniques. The publication is available online at: <http://www.tiesmagazine.org>.

TSM Connection Activities

Technology Education; 144 Smyth Hall, Virginia Tech, Blacksburg, VA 24061-0432; Phone: 540-231-6480

These 11 activities designed to integrate the instruction of math, science, and technology at the middle school level were developed through the Technology, Science, and Mathematics Integration Project (TSM). The activities challenge students to design, construct, and test solutions to real-world problems. The TSM units encourage team teaching and include detailed suggestions for math, science, and technology teachers. Details can be found at: <http://teched.vt.edu/TechEd/HTML/Research/TSMOverview1.html>.

World in Motion

SAE: World in Motion; 400 Commonwealth Drive, Warrendale, PA 15096-0001; Phone: 877-606-7323; Email: awim@sae.org

Students working in "engineering design teams" explore physics through a series of activities, including designing boats, cars, and steel can rovers. Developed by the Society of Automotive Engineers in 1990, this curriculum kit provides a physical science supplement for grades 4, 5, and 6.

A World in Motion: The Design Experience is a multidisciplinary curriculum for grades 7 and 8. Teachers who enlist the support of engineers are eligible to receive free curriculum kits that includes a teacher's manual, manipulatives, and promotional materials. Details are available at: <www.sae.org/students/awim.htm>.

Standards and Related Publications

Benchmarks for Science Literacy

Benchmarks for Science Literacy is the AAAS Project 2061 statement of what all students should know and be able to do in science, mathematics, and technology by the end of grades 2, 5, 8, and 12. *Benchmarks* provides educators with sequences of specific learning goals that can be used to design a core curriculum. The nature of technology and the designed world benchmarks relate directly to technological literacy. *Benchmarks* can be found online at: <www.project2061.org/tools/benchol/bolframe.htm>.

Massachusetts Curriculum Frameworks

Massachusetts Department of Education; 350 Main Street, Malden, MA 02148-5023; Phone: 781-338-3460; Email: blibby@doe.mass.edu

The Massachusetts Department of Education has created the country's first statewide K-12 curriculum framework that explicitly includes engineering. A complete copy of the framework is available online in PDF format at: <www.doe.mass.edu/frameworks/default.html>.

National Science Education Standards

The National Science Education Standards (NSES) outline what scientifically literate students should know, understand, and be able to do at different grade levels. Standards on science and technology focus on establishing connections between the natural and designed worlds and developing decision-making abilities. The NSES can be found online at: <www.nap.edu/readingroom/books/nses/html/contents.html>.

Principles and Standards for School Mathematics

Principles and Standards for School Mathematics is a set of comprehensive goals in mathematics for all K-12 students. Developed by the National Council of Teachers of Mathematics, these standards include probability, problem solving, and making connections to other subject areas, such as science and technology. The website address is: <standards.nctm.org>.

Standards for Technological Literacy: Content for the Study of Technology

International Technology Education Association; 1914 Association Drive, Suite 201, Reston, VA 20191; Phone: 703-860-2100; Email: itea@iris.org

This ITEA report presents 20 standards of what technologically literate K-12 students should know and be able to do in five general areas, as well as several benchmarks for specific grade levels. ITEA is currently developing a series of curriculum guides to assist teachers and other educators to implement the standards. The website address is: <www.iteawww.org/TAA/STLstds.htm>.

Organizations of Interest

Association for Career and Technical Education and EdGate

1410 King Street, Alexandria, VA 22314; Phone: 800-826-9972; Email: acte@acteonline.org; Website: <www.acteonline.org>

The Association for Career and Technical Education (ACTE), formerly the American Vocational Association, is the largest national education association dedicated to preparing youths and adults for careers. Founded in 1926, ACTE members are teachers, administrators, guidance counselors, university professors, state/local employees, and students in subject areas ranging from business to health care.

Association of Science-Technology Centers

1025 Vermont Avenue, NW, Suite 500, Washington, DC 20005-3516; Phone: 202-783-7200; Email: info@astc.org; Website: <www.astc.org>

The Association of Science-Technology Centers (ASTC) is an organization of informal education centers and museums dedicated to furthering the public understanding of science. Founded in 1973, the members of ASTC include science-technology centers and science museums, nature centers, aquariums, planetariums, zoos, botanical gardens, space theaters, and children's museums.

The Center for Engineering Education Outreach

Tufts University School of Engineering; 105 Anderson Hall, Medford, MA 02155; Phone: 617-627-5888; Email: martha.cyr@tufts.edu; Website: <www.ceeo.tufts.edu/default.asp>

The Center for Engineering Educational Outreach at Tufts University is dedicated to bringing engineering into the K-12 classroom. Using the model of engineering design projects, the center coordinates the work of experts in engineering and education with teachers to create engineering-based curricula.

Center for Occupational Research and Development

P.O. Box 21689, Waco, TX 76702-1689; Phone: 254-772-8756; Email: webmaster@cord.org; Website: <www.cord.org>

The Center for Occupational Research and Development (CORD) is a national nonprofit organization that promotes innovations in education to prepare students for careers and higher education. CORD assists educators in secondary schools and colleges through new curricula, teaching strategies, professional development, and partnerships with community leaders, families, and employers.

International Technology Education Association

1914 Association Drive, Suite 201, Reston, VA 20191-1539; Phone: 703-860-2100; Email: itea@iris.org; Website: <www.iteawww.org/index.html>

The goal of ITEA, the professional organization of technology teachers, is to promote overall technological literacy by supporting the teaching of technology by professional, well-educated teachers. ITEA developed the *Standards for Technological Literacy* and supports the publication of *Technology Teacher*, a magazine for technology education professionals, and the *Journal of Technology Education*, a scholarly publication focused on technology education research, philosophy, and theory.

Jerome and Dorothy Lemelson Center for the Study of Invention and Innovation

National Museum of American History, Room 1016, Smithsonian Institution, Washington, DC 20560-0604; Phone: 202-357-1593; Email: LemCen@nmah.si.edu; Website: <www.si.edu/lemelson>

The Jerome and Dorothy Lemelson Center for the Study of Invention and Innovation documents, interprets, and disseminates information about inventions and innovations. The center supports programs and events to encourage young people to be inventive and to recognize the role of invention and innovation in U.S. history. The Lemelson Center, housed at the Smithsonian Institution's National Museum of American History, has extensive resources for teachers, students, and others.

Junior Engineering Technical Society

1420 King Street, Suite 405, Alexandria, VA 22314-2794; Phone: 703-548-5387; Email: jetsinfo@jets.org; Website: <www.jets.org>

Junior Engineering Technical Society (JETS) sponsors competitions, programs, and other activities and provides educational materials about the world of engineering showing how math and science are used to solve technological problems that have social, political, and economic effects. JETS sponsors the Tests of Engineering Aptitude, Mathematics, and Science (TEAMS) and the National Engineering Design Challenge (NEDC), and the National Engineering Aptitude Search+ (NEAS+), a self-administered academic survey that enables students to determine their current level of preparation in applied mathematics, science, and reasoning.

The Loka Institute

P.O. Box 355, Amherst, MA 01004-0355; Phone: 413-559-5860; Email: loka@loka.org; Website: <www.loka.org>

The Loka Institute is a nonprofit research and advocacy organization concerned with the social, political, and environmental repercussions of research, science, and technology. Since 1987, the Loka Institute has created and/or supported programs to promote more informed science and technology policy by making it more responsive to social and environmental concerns. Loka strives to increase opportunities for individual, grassroots, and public-interest group involvement in science and technology decision making.

NACME, Inc.

Empire State Building; 350 Fifth Avenue, Suite 2212; New York, NY 10118-2299; Phone: 212-279-2626; Website: <www.nacme.org>

The National Action Council for Minorities in Engineering, Inc. (NACME), provides leadership and support for national efforts to increase the participation of African Americans, American Indians, and Latinos in engineering, and technology-, math-, and science-based careers.

National Science Resources Center

955 L'Enfant Plaza, SW, Suite 8400, Washington, DC 20560-0952; Phone: 202-287-2063; Email: nsrcsite@si.edu; Website: <www.si.edu/nsrc/default.htm>

The National Science Resources Center (NSRC), operated jointly by the National Academies and the Smithsonian Institution, is dedicated to improving the teaching of science. NSRC is a clearinghouse for information about exemplary teaching resources and develops and disseminates science curriculum materials for elementary classrooms. The center also sponsors outreach activities to help school districts develop and sustain hands-on science programs.

National Skill Standards Board

1441 L Street, NW, Suite 9000, Washington, DC 20005-3512; Phone: 202-254-8628; Email: information@nssb.org; Website: <www.nssb.org>

The National Skill Standards Board is a coalition of community, business, labor, education, and civil rights leaders. The board is building a national voluntary system of skill standards, assessment, and certification.

Project 2061

AAAS; 1200 New York Ave., NW, Washington, DC 20005; Phone: 202-326-6666; Email: project2061@aaas.org; Website: <project2061.aaas.org>

Project 2061 of the American Association for the Advancement of Science is a long-term initiative to reform K-12 science education. The project is creating coordinated reform tools and services in the form of books, CD-ROMs, and online resources. Established in 1985, Project 2061 provides support to enable all Americans to become literate in science, mathematics, and technology. A 1989 publication, *Science for All Americans*, provided recommendations for what all students should know, and be able to do, in science, mathematics, and technology by the time they graduate from high school.

Salvadori Center

c/o City College, Y Building 308A, 135th Street & Convent Avenue, New York, NY 10031-9198; Phone: 212-650-5497; Email: thecenter@salvadori.org; Website: <www.salvadori.org/index.html>

The Salvadori Middle School Program (SMSP) in New York City, the core program of the Salvadori Center, offers teacher training and support to improve student academic performance and critical thinking skills. Fully integrated, hands-on projects focusing on the built environment help students learn math, science, and the humanities while developing an appreciation for the aesthetics, history, and practice of engineering. Teachers from participating middle schools attend a summer institute and meet regularly to continue sharing their experiences in implementing the SMSP.

Society for the History of Technology

Department of the History of Science, 216B Ames Hall, Johns Hopkins University, Baltimore, MD 21218; Phone: 410-516-8349; Email: shot@jhu.edu; Website: <http://shot.press.jhu.edu>

Society for the History of Technology (SHOT) is an interdisciplinary organization concerned with the history of technological devices and processes and the relationship of technology to science, politics, social change, the arts and humanities, and economics. SHOT members include practicing scientists and engineers, anthropologists, librarians, political scientists, and economists. The organization publishes a regular newsletter and *Technology and Culture*, a quarterly journal.

Society of Women Engineers

230 East Ohio Street, Suite 400, Chicago, IL 60611-3265; Phone: 312-596-5223; Email: hq@swe.org; Website: <www.swe.org>

The Society of Women Engineers (SWE) encourages women to achieve their full potential in careers as engineers and leaders, increases public awareness of the engineering profession, and demonstrates the value of diversity. Like many other engineering societies, SWE supports an active network of volunteers who go into classrooms and work with after-school programs to interest students in math, science, and technology.

Contests and Awards

BEST

Boosting Engineering, Science, and Technology; Email: bestinc@bestinc.org

The Boosting Engineering, Science, and Technology (BEST) competition exposes middle and high school students to the concepts of engineering and technology through a robotics design challenge. Teams have 6 weeks to design and build prototypes of a remote-controlled robot that can accomplish a specific task. Competitors advance from local events to a regional play-off and championship. Details can be found at: <www.bestinc.org>.

Craftsman/NSTA Young Inventors Award

National Science Teachers Association; 1840 Wilson Boulevard, Arlington, VA 22201-3000; Phone: 888-494-4994; Email: younginventors@nsta.org

The Craftsman/NSTA Young Inventors Awards Program challenges students to use their creativity and imagination, along with their science, technology, and mechanical ability, to invent or modify a tool. The competition runs from late August to mid-March with separate divisions for grades 2 through 5 and 6 through 8. Details can be found online at: <www.nsta.org/programs/craftsman/>.

Draper Prize

National Academy of Engineering; 2101 Constitution Avenue, NW, Washington, DC 20418; Phone: 202-334-1237

The Charles Stark Draper Prize is a preeminent award for engineering achievement. This annual prize honors an engineer or group of engineers whose accomplishments have significantly improved the quality of life, improved people's ability to live freely and comfortably, and/or permitted access to information. The $500,000 award is intended to increase public awareness of the contributions of engineers and technology to the welfare and freedom of humanity. Details can found at: <www.nae.edu>.

FIRST LEGO League

200 Bedford Street, Manchester, NH 03101; Phone: 800-871-8326; Email: FLL@usfirst.org

Teams of 9- to 14-year-olds use LEGO bricks, sensors, motors, and gears to construct and program fully autonomous robots capable of completing different missions while maneuvering around a 4-foot-by-8-foot playing field. Teams are mentored by adults or sometimes high school students who competed in the FIRST Robotics Competition. Details about the contest, including past challenges, can be found online at: <www.legomindstorms.com/fll>.

FIRST Robotics Competition

200 Bedford Street, Manchester, NH 03101; Phone: 800-871-8326; Email: frc@usfirst.org

The FIRST Robotics Competition is a national engineering contest for high school students in which student teams work with engineers from business and universities to brainstorm, design, construct, and test "champion robots." The competition, which takes place over a period of 6 weeks, kicks off in January and culminates with the national championship in April. Details are available at: <www.usfirst.org/robotics/index.html>.

Future City Competition™

1420 King Street, Alexandria, VA 22314; Phone: 703-684-2852; Email: eweek@nspe.org

Working with a teacher and an engineer, student teams design a future city using a computer program and then build a scale model of a section of their city. Teams must also write a 500-word essay on a specific engineering topic and make an oral presentation of their work. The winners of regional contests compete at the national level for awards sponsored by various organizations and businesses. Details of the contest, sponsored by National Engineers Week, can be found online at: <www.futurecity.org>.

Future Problem Solving Program

Future Problem Solving Program; 2028 Regency Road, Lexington, KY 40503; Phone: 800-256-1499; Email: FPSolve@aol.com

The Future Problem Solving Program (FPSP) emphasizes using creative problem-solving skills to address a variety of anticipated problems. The program features both competitive and noncompetitive activities. Under the guidance of teachers/coaches, teams of four students in grades 4 through 12 explore challenges and propose action plans to address complex societal problems. The program is designed to be used in the regular classroom to introduce students to creative problem solving in a hands-on, nonthreatening environment. Details of the program can be found at: <www.fpsp.org>.

Gordon Prize for Innovation in Engineering and Technology Education

National Academy of Engineering; 2101 Constitution Avenue, NW, Washington, DC 20418; Phone: 202-334-1237

 The National Academy of Engineering Bernard M. Gordon Prize is a biennial cash award of $500,000 given to an individual or small group of individuals for a specific project/program or for a body of work over a period of years. The prize is intended to encourage improvements of engineering and technology education relevant to the practice of engineering, the maintenance of a strong, diverse engineering workforce, innovation and inventiveness, and the promotion of technology development. Details can found at: <www.nae.edu/awards>.

Intel International Science and Engineering Fair

Science Service; 1719 N Street, NW, Washington, DC 20036; Phone: 202-785-2255; Email: sciedu@sciserv.org

 The Intel International Science and Engineering Fair (ISEF) is the world's largest precollege science competition. Young scientists from around the world come together in May of each year to share ideas, showcase cutting-edge science projects, and compete for more than $3 million in awards and scholarships. Rules and guidelines, as well as science and engineering resources, are available on the ISEF website at: <www.sciserv.org/isef/index.asp>.

Lemelson-MIT Awards

Massachusetts Institute of Technology; 77 Massachusetts Avenue, Room E 60-324, Cambridge, MA 02139; Phone: 617-253-3352; Email: invent@mit.edu

 The Lemelson-MIT Prize is a $500,000 award presented to an American inventor-innovator for outstanding inventiveness and creativity in the field of science, medicine, engineering, or entrepreneurship. Annual awards are also presented to outstanding college and high school innovators. Invention Dimension, the program's website (web.mit.edu/invent), includes an "inventor of the week" feature and extensive links and other resources.

National Engineering Design Challenge

Junior Engineering Technical Society; 1420 King Street, Suite 405, Alexandria, VA 22314-2794; Phone: 703-548-5387; Email: jetsinfo@jets.org.

 National Engineering Design Challenge (NEDC) encourages

teams of high school students to work with engineer advisers to design, fabricate, and demonstrate a working solution to a social need. NEDC is a cooperative program between Junior Engineering Technical Society, the National Society of Professional Engineers, and the National Talent Network. Teams present their solutions before a panel of judges at a regional competition, and the winners advance to the national finals held in Washington, D.C., during National Engineers Week, in February. Details of the contest can be found at: <www.jets.org/nedc.htm>.

Odyssey of the Mind

Odyssey of the Mind Program; c/o Creative Competitions Inc., 1325 Rt. 130 South, Suite F, Gloucester City, NJ 08030; Phone: 856-456-7776; Email: info@odysseyofthemind.com

This international program encourages creative problem solving by challenging students in a variety of areas, from building mechanical devices to interpreting literary classics. Teams of five to seven students compete in four grade-level divisions. Each year five new problems are presented to be solved over a period of weeks or months. At competitions, teams present their solution to a "long-run" problem; they are then given an on-the-spot "spontaneous" problem to solve. Details and practice problems can be found online at <www.odysseyofthemind.com>.

RI/SME Student Robotic Engineering Challenge

Society of Manufacturing Engineers; One SME Drive, P.O. Box 930, Dearborn, MI 48121-0930; Phone: 313-271-1500; Email: cartkat@sme.org

The RI/SME is a competition for middle school through college students that tests knowledge of the manufacturing process as demonstrated through robotics and automation contests. Teams from middle and high schools, community colleges, and universities compete in 14 different categories. Students are judged on their application of manufacturing principles and their ability to solve manufacturing-related problems through a team approach. Details can be found at: <www.sme.org>.

Toshiba/NSTA Exploravision Awards

1840 Wilson Boulevard, Arlington, VA 22201-3000; Phone: 800-EXPLOR-9 or 703-243-7100; Email: exploravision@nsta.org

The Toshiba/NSTA Exploravision Awards encourage students to combine the tools of science with their own imaginations to create a vision of future technologies. Teams of two, three, or four students simulate research and development teams and, with the guidance of a team coach and mentor (optional), select a technology or an aspect of a technology relevant to their lives. They then imagine what the technology will be like 20 years from now and convey their vision to others through written descriptions and five graphics simulating web pages. Details can be found at: <www.toshiba.com/tai/exploravision>.

APPENDIX B
Committee and Staff Biographies

Committee on Technological Literacy

A. THOMAS YOUNG, *chair,* is a member of the National Academy of Engineering and retired executive vice president of Lockheed Martin. Mr. Young was previously president and chief operating officer of Martin Marietta Corporation. Prior to joining industry, Mr. Young worked for 21 years at the National Aeronautics and Space Administration (NASA), where he directed the Goddard Space Flight Center, was deputy director of the Ames Research Center, directed the Planetary Program in the Office of Space Science at NASA headquarters, and was mission director for the Project Viking Mars landing program. He has been a member of several National Research Council committees, including the Office of Science and Engineering Personnel Advisory Committee and the Committee on Supply Chain Integration: New Roles and Challenges for Small and Medium-Sized Companies.

PAUL ALLAN has been working on teacher professional development at Pacific Science Center in Seattle, Washington, for the past 2 years. Before that, he taught physics, mathematics, and technology courses at Colony High School in Palmer, Alaska, for 9 years. A classroom teacher for 20 years, Mr. Allan received his M.S. in science education from Columbia University Teachers College and his B.A. in biology. Mr. Allan has participated in the Dartmouth Project for Teaching Engineering Problem Solving and has served as president of the Alaska Council of Teachers of Mathematics. Mr. Allan's recent awards include the 1996 Teacher of the Year at Colony High School, 1994 Presidential Award for Excellence in Science Teaching, and 1999 Distinguished Physics Teacher from Alaska by the American Physical Society.

WILLIAM ANDERS, retired chairman of General Dynamics, was a U.S. Air Force fighter pilot and engineer until being selected as a NASA astronaut. In 1968, he flew with Frank Borman and James Lovell aboard the Apollo 8 lunar mission, the first spacecraft to leave the Earth and orbit the moon. From 1969 to 1973 he was the executive secretary of the National Aeronautics and Space Council, and from 1973 to 1975 he was chairman of the Nuclear Regulatory Commission. From 1976 to 1977 he was U.S. Ambassador to Norway. Mr. Anders is a member of the National Academy of Engineering, a trustee of the Battelle Memorial Institute, and a member of the board of the Center for Occupational Research and Development, an organization that develops comprehensive tech-prep programs designed to enable students to make a successful transition from school to work.

TAFT H. BROOME, JR. is professor of civil engineering at Howard University. During his 29-year career at Howard, Dr. Broome has been department chair and chair of the University Senate. In 1985, he received his M.S. in science, technology, and society from Rensselaer Polytechnic Institute. Dr. Broome has served in leadership positions of major national organizations, including the American Association for the Advancement of Science, American Society for Engineering Education, and the National Association for Science, Technology, and Society. Among his many publications is "Race and the Information Super Highway: Implications for a Participatory Democracy," a chapter in *The Information Society and the Black Community* (Greenwood, forthcoming). He is a member of the board of directors of Women in Engineering Program Advocates Network and of the National Academy of Engineering's Committee on Engineering Education.

JONATHAN R. COLE is provost and dean of faculties at Columbia University, as well as the John Mitchell Mason Professor at the university. Dr. Cole has spent much of his academic career studying the social aspects of science and technology and developing the sociology of science. He has published widely on many subjects, including the system of social stratification in science; the reward system of science; the place of women in the scientific community; the growth of knowledge; the measurement of the quality of scientific work; the communications system in science; the social construction of medical facts; and the peer review system in science, particularly at the National Science Foundation. His recent publications have focused on the structure of the research university and the new digital media and intellectual property. Dr. Cole has had a long-standing interest in questions of scientific and technological literacy. He has been a Guggenheim fellow, fellow of the Center for Advanced Study in the Behavior Sciences, and been elected to the American Academy of Arts and Sciences, among other honors. He has served on many advisory boards and committees of the National Academies and the National Science Foundation.

RODNEY L. CUSTER, chair of the Department of Industrial Technology at Illinois State University, is a national leader in technology education and chair of the Secondary Standards Development Team for the International Technology Education Association's initiative to develop K-12 standards in technology education. Dr. Custer is a member of the National Research Council's Committee on Teacher Preparation in Science, Mathematics, and Technology Education: Integrating Research Recommendations and the Realities of Practice, and the National Academy of Engineering's Committee on Engineering Education.

GOÉRY DELACÔTE is a renowned scientist, science educator, and public servant who joined the Exploratorium as executive director in February 1991. He is currently on leave from the University of Paris, where he is professor of physics. Dr. Delacôte has a Ph.D. in solid state physics from the École Normale Supérieure and has been involved in science and science education since the outset of his career. From 1982 to 1991, Dr. Delacôte was the director of the Science and Technology Information Division of the Centre National de la Recherche Scientifique (CNRS). He has also been a member of the Board of Trustees of the Bibliothèque de France, the new National Library of France (1989 to 1993). Dr. Delacôte served on the National Committee on Science Education Standards and Assessment of the National Research Council, which issued K-12 science education standards in September 1995. As executive secretary of the Exploratorium, Dr. Delacôte has implemented a new approach combining exhibits, networking, and teacher education to create a public laboratory on learning with outreach to a large audience of scientists, artists, educators, children, and families. Under his leadership, many Exploratorium partnerships have been established in the United States and abroad.

DENICE DENTON is professor of electrical engineering and dean of engineering at the University of Washington, Seattle. Prior to her current position, she was professor of electrical engineering at the University of Wisconsin-Madison. In addition to serving on several visiting committees for the National Science Foundation (NSF) Directorate for Engineering, she has been involved in many activities in the NSF Directorate for Education and Human Resources (EHR). Most recently, she served on the EHR Advisory Committee, which was responsible for a major review of undergraduate education. She also chaired the National Research Council Board on Engineering Education.

PAUL DE VORE is president of PWD Associates, a consulting company which he founded. Prior to that, Dr. De Vore was professor and chair, Department of Technology Education, West Virginia University; research associate (history of technology), Smithsonian Institution; and director, Division of Education and Training, National Technology Transfer Center. Among his publications are a monograph, *Technology and the New Liberal Arts* (University of Northern Iowa, 1976), which explores the relation between the study of technology as a discipline and the study of technology as part of a liberal education, and several books, including *Technology: An Intellectual Discipline* (American Industrial Arts Association, 1964); *Structure and Content: Foundations for Curriculum Development* (American Industrial Arts Association, 1968; reprinted 1973), which contributed to the establishment of technology education as a national movement; and *Technology: An Introduction* (Davis Publications, 1980), a leading college textbook and reference. He is also the editor of *Introduction to Transportation* (Davis Publications, 1983) and coauthor of *Creativity in the Technologies* (Davis Publications, 1989).

KAREN FALKENBERG is currently a full-time doctoral candidate at Emory University; her dissertation will focus on creativity, innovation, and education. Most recently, she was the program manager for the Elementary Science Education Partners Program (ESEP), a five-year

NSF-funded science education reform project based in Atlanta, Georgia. ESEP was a collaborative effort between eight institutions of higher education in the metropolitan Atlanta area and the urban Atlanta Public School District. ESEP provided professional development, classroom materials, and undergraduate science partners to more than 1,600 elementary teachers, and the program influenced the science instruction for more than 35,000 elementary students. Ms. Falkenberg is an international education consultant, a member of the Southeastern Regional Vision for Education Leadership Academy for Science and Mathematics, and a mentor for the WestEd National Academy for Science and Mathematics Education Leadership. She has served on the NSF's teacher enhancement panel, has been a faculty member for the National Science Resources Center's Leadership Academy for Science Education Reform, and was a featured classroom teacher in case studies of prominent U.S. innovations in science, math, and technology education. Ms. Falkenberg worked as a research engineer and taught high school before entering the field of science education reform.

SHELAGH A. GALLAGHER is assistant professor of education at the University of North Carolina, Charlotte, where she also directs a U.S. Department of Education project, P-BLISS (Problem-Based Learning in the Social Sciences). She has spent many years conducting training and research on problem-based learning and studying the characteristics of gifted adolescents and gender differences in the development and expression of talent. Dr. Gallagher has served as director of measurement for the Longitudinal Study of American Youth at the Chicago Academy of Science and director of research and assessment at the Illinois Mathematics and Science Academy. At the College of William and Mary, she was project manager for the Javits Science Curriculum Project, which included a review of science curricula and the production of six problem-based science units.

JOYCE GARDELLA, principal of Gardella & Associates, a strategic marketing consulting firm, has expertise in marketing science and technology concepts and programs. Prior to launching her own business, Ms. Gardella was vice president for marketing at the Museum of Science in Boston and before that marketing director at the Museum of Science & Industry and Brookfield Zoo, both in Chicago.

DAVID T. HARRISON, vice president of educational programs at Seminole Community College in Sanford, Florida, is responsible for student learning in the liberal arts, sciences, business and information technology, health professions, criminal justice and public service, and other professional and technological fields. He also oversees an alternative high school, adult basic education programs, and language programs for international students. Dr. Harrison has worked extensively on lifelong learning opportunities, and on economic, workforce, and community development issues.

PAUL HOFFMAN is working on a book on the history of flying machines before the Wright Brothers. A former president of Encyclopedia Britannica and editor in chief of *Discover* magazine, he has a long history of involvement in communicating science and technology to the public. Mr. Hoffman has been a special science correspondent for "Good Morning America" and has appeared on CNN, "ABC News," and "The Charlie Rose Show." He has written for many national magazines, including *The New Yorker*, *The Atlantic Monthly*, *The New York Times Magazine*, *Smithsonian*, and *Business Week*, and was the first winner of the National Magazine Award for Feature Writing. He has written 10 books, including the international bestseller, *The Man Who Loved Only Numbers: The Story of Paul Erdos and the Search for Mathematical Truth* (Hyperion, 1998).

JONDEL (J.D.) HOYE is president of Keep the Change, a workforce development consulting firm. Ms. Hoye is the immediate past director of the National School-to-Work Office, a joint initiative of the U.S. Departments of Labor and Education. Prior to her work in the federal government, Ms. Hoye was associate superintendent of the Oregon Department of Education and Office of Community College Services. In that position, she was responsible for professional, vocational, and technical education statewide.

THOMAS P. HUGHES is Mellon Professor Emeritus, University of Pennsylvania, and a distinguished visiting professor at MIT, a visiting professor at Stanford University, and a visiting professor at the Royal Institute of Technology in Stockholm. Dr. Hughes, who did his graduate work in European history at the University of Virginia, has published books on American and European history that pay especial attention to the history of modern technology, science, and culture. His publications include two books about the nature of technological and social change: *Networks of Power: Electrification of Western Society, 1880–1930* (Johns Hopkins University Press, 1983) and *Elmer Sperry: Inventor and Engineer* (Johns Hopkins University Press, 1971). Both books won Dexter Prizes for outstanding books in the history of technology. *American Genesis: A Century of Invention and Technological Enthusiasm, 1870–1970* (Penguin USA, 1990) was one of the three finalists for the 1990 Pulitzer Prize in history. His most recent book is *Rescuing Prometheus* (Pantheon Books, 1998), which focuses on managing the creation of large technological systems. Dr. Hughes has been chairman of the Department of the History and Sociology of Science, University of Pennsylvania; the NASA History Advisory Committee; and the U.S. National Committee for the History and Philosophy of Science. He is a history consultant for ABC television, WGBH television, and the Sloan Foundation and has been a member of the Advisory Council to the Secretary of the Smithsonian Institution. He chaired the National Research Council Committee on Innovations in Computing and Communications: Lessons from History.

MAE JEMISON was the first woman of color to travel into space when she flew on the space shuttle *Endeavor* in 1992. Since resigning from NASA, Jemison has founded The Jemison Group, a technology design and consulting company in Houston that focuses on the beneficial integration of science and technology into everyday life. Jemison is also a professor of environmental studies and director of the Jemison Institute for Advancing Technology in Developing Countries at Dartmouth College. The institute promotes sustainable development—improving the quality of life without compromising the opportunities for future generations to grow and prosper. Jemison speaks nationally on the importance of education, adult responsibility, and universal science literacy. She established The Earth We Share™, an international science camp for 12- to 16-year-olds that builds critical thinking and problem-solving skills through an experiential curriculum. She also serves as Bayer Corporation's National Science Literacy Advocate. Jemison is an engineer and physician, and the author of a young adult autobiography, *Finding Where the Wind Goes: Moments From My Life* (Scholastic, 2001).

F. JAMES RUTHERFORD is education advisor to the executive officer of the American Association for the Advancement of Science (AAAS) and has extensive experience in planning and overseeing efforts to reform the U.S. K-12 education system. At AAAS, he has been responsible for several national initiatives, including Science Resources for Schools, Challenge of the Unknown, the National Forum for School Science, and Science Seminars for Teachers, and for several publications, including *Science Education News*, the annual *Science Education Directory*, the annual *This Year in School Science*, and *Science Education in Global Perspective*. As initiator and director of Project 2061, he headed the nation's most prominent, long-term, comprehensive effort to promote nationwide reform in science, mathematics, and technology education. Prior to joining AAAS, Dr. Rutherford served in two federal agencies. In 1977, he was appointed by President Carter to be assistant director of the National Science Foundation responsible for all science, mathematics, and engineering education programs, preschool through postdoctoral, and for federal programs to improve the public understanding of science. When the new U.S. Department of Education was launched, President Carter appointed him assistant secretary for research and improvement, a position that included responsibility for the National Institute of Education, the National Center for Educational Statistics, the Fund for the Improvement of Post-Secondary Education, and federal programs supporting libraries and the development of educational technologies. Earlier, Rutherford was professor of science education at Harvard University and at New York University, and earlier still, a high school science teacher in California.

KATHRYN C. THORNTON is professor of technology, culture, and communication and director of the Center for Science, Mathematics, and Engineering Education at the University of Virginia in Charlottesville. The center is an interdisciplinary office coordinating the activities of the university's engineering school, Curry School of Education, College of Arts and Sciences, and Office of the Vice President for Research and Public Service. Previously, for 12 years Dr. Thornton served as an astronaut based at the Johnson Space Center, where her duties included participating in space missions and heading the Education Working Group. She is a member of the National Research Council Aeronautics and Space Engineering Board.

ROBERT TINKER is founder, president, and chairman of the Concord Consortium in Concord, Massachusetts. For more than 20 years, he has conducted pioneering work in constructivist approaches to education, particularly novel uses of educational technology in science and mathematics. Prior to founding the Concord Consortium, Dr. Tinker was director of TERC (formerly the Technical Education Research Center), where he developed the idea of equipping computers with probes for real-time measurements and of using the Internet for collaborative student data sharing and investigations. Dr. Tinker has taught college physics for more than 10 years.

Project Staff

GREG PEARSON is a program officer with the National Academy of Engineering (NAE), where he directs the academy's efforts related to technological literacy. In this capacity, Mr. Pearson most recently served as the responsible staff officer for the Committee on Technological Literacy, a joint project of the NAE and the National Research Council. He also oversaw a review of national K-12 content standards for the study of technology developed by the International Technology Education Association. He has worked collaboratively with colleagues within and outside the National Academies on a variety of projects involving K-12 science, mathematics, technology, and engineering education and the public understanding of engineering and science. Pearson has a B.A. in biology from Swarthmore College and an M.A. in journalism from The American University.

ROBERT POOL is a freelance writer based in Tallahassee, Florida, who specializes in science and technology. He has written for a number of magazines, including *Science, Nature, Discover, New Scientist,* and *Technology Review* and is the author of three books, including *Beyond Engineering: How Society Shapes Technology* (Oxford University Press, 1997). He was also a writing consultant for the International Technology Education Association *Standards for Technological Literacy* (ITEA, 2000).

Index

Black persons, 42, 43, 129, 138, 143
Boosting Engineering, Science, and
        Technology, 131-132
Britain, *see* United Kingdom
British School Examinations
        Assessment Council, 69
Building Big, 121
Buildings, Bridges, and Tunnels, 116

C

Canada, 68-69, 70
Carl D. Perkins Vocational Education
        Act, 82
Center for Engineering Education
        Outreach, 128
Center for Occupational Research and
        Development, 82-83, 128
Children Designing and Engineering
        Project, 121-122
City Technology Project, 122
Colleges and universities, 7, 84-88, 124,
        128, 133
    see also Teacher education
    museums and science centers, 89
    public decision making, 95, 112
Commission on Achieving Necessary
        Skills, 41
Competency, technical, *see* Technical
        competency
Computer technology, 4, 5-6, 13-15,
        58-59, 133
    see also Internet
    adult literacy, 64
    climate models, 14
    curriculum standards, 81
    digital divide, 42-44, 45, 61, 138
    Global Positioning System, 41
    mass media coverage, 67, 90-91
    overemphasis on, 58-63
    primary and secondary education,
        5-6, 44
        digital divide, 42-44, 45, 61, 138
        overemphasis on, 58-59
    teaching with technology *vs* teaching
        about technology, 6, 58-59
Congress, *see* Legislation; Office of
        Technology Assessment
Consensus conferences, 39, 95, 97
Constructive technology assessment, 96,
        144-145

Consumer decision making, 3, 16, 25
    automobile air bags, 22, 26-29, 65
    genetically modified organisms, 14,
        18, 26, 29-32
Contests and awards, 98
    students, 93-94, 131-136
    teachers, 10, 113-114
Cost and cost-benefit factors, 4, 20
    see also Risk assessment
    automobile air bags, 27
    Boston Central Artery and Tunnel,
        37-40
    California energy crisis, 36
    engineering process, 52
Council for Basic Education, 56
Council of State Governments, 62
Council on Technology Teacher
        Education, 87-88
Craftsman/NSTA Young Inventors
        Award, 132
Cultural factors, 4, 16, 23, 81, 118, 120
    see also Political factors; Social factors
    religious issues, 117, 119
Curriculum and instructional materials
        development, 2, 77-80, 91-92,
        104, 105, 109, 113
    biomedical sciences, 78, 79, 81
    Department of Education, 8-9, 105,
        107
    federal government involvement, 9,
        82, 83
    inventive programs, 10, 105
    National Science Foundation, 6-7,
        8-9, 56, 57, 82, 105, 107, 123,
        141
    national standards, 9, 78-79, 80, 104,
        105, 106-108, 126-127
    postsecondary education, 85
    resources for technological literacy
        summarized, 121-125, 128-
        129, 130
    state standards, 8, 9, 126
    technician preparation/vocational
        education, 82-83
    textbooks, 77-78, 105-106

D

Danish Board of Technology, 95, 111
Decision making, 3-4, 8, 25-35, 45,
        94-98, 103-104, 110-113
    see also Problem solving

Ethnicity, *see* Race/ethnicity
European Awareness Scenario
    Workshop, 95-96
European Union
    genetically modified organisms, 30
    public opinion/knowledge polls, 69
    urban areas, public participation in
        decision making, 95-96
The Existential Pleasures of Engineering,
    117

F

Federal government, 2, 7, 63, 71, 84
    see also Funding; Legislation; *terms
        beginning "Department of..."*
    automobile air bags, 27
    Boston Central Artery and Tunnel,
        38-40
    defense applications, 41
    genetically modified organisms, 30
    infrastructure projects, public
        education, 9
    National Aeronautics and Space
        Administration, 57, 61, 67,
        82, 124, 137, 138, 143, 144
    primary and secondary education, 8,
        82, 83, 104-105, 107, 130
    teacher awards, 10, 113-114
    public participation in decision
        making, 7, 94-95, 97-98,
        110-112
    vocational education, 83
Federal Highway Administration, 39-40
Fellowship programs, 10, 111-112
FIRST LEGO League, 132
FIRST Robotics Competition, 93, 94,
    133
Food science, genetically modified
    organisms, 14, 18, 26, 29-32
Foreign countries, *see* International
    perspectives
Foundations, 9, 91-93, 95, 111-112
    see also National Science Foundation
Funding, 9, 58, 61, 62, 86
    see also Contests and awards;
        Department of Education;
        National Science Foundation
    civic decision making, 94-95
    committee study sponsorship, *vii*, 2,
        12
    fellowship programs, 10, 112-113

primary and secondary education,
    6-7, 8-9, 56-57, 109
    computer technology, 58-59, 61
    curricula and instructional
        materials, 6-7, 8-9, 56, 57, 82,
        91-92, 105, 109, 123
    school-to-work partnerships, 84
    student awards, 93-94
    teacher awards, 10, 113-114
    teacher training, 59-60, 91-92
Future City Competition, 94, 133
Future Problem Solving Program, 133

G

Gallup Organization, 64, 68, 71
Gender factors, 123, 141
    automobile air bags, 28
    Society of Women Engineers, 131
    student attitudes toward technology,
        63
Genetics
    genetically modified organisms, 14,
        18, 26, 29-32, 67
    public participation in decision
        making, 95
Gordon Prize for Innovation in
    Engineering and Technology
    Education, 134
Government, 52
    see also Federal government; Political
        factors; State government
    civic decision making, 3-4, 7, 11, 12,
        21, 22, 23, 36-40, 65-66,
        70-71, 86-87, 90, 94-98.
        103-104, 110-111
    fellowship programs, 10, 111-112
    leadership, 3-4, 9, 12, 16, 26, 70.
        111-112, 114
Great Britain, *see* United Kingdom
The Great Idea Finder, 117
Greatest Achievements of the 20th Century,
    117

H

Handbook of Science and Technology, 86
Health and safety issues, 48, 52, 67
    see also Biomedical sciences
    automobile air bags, 26-29

J

Jefferson, Thomas, 11
Jerome and Dorothy Lemelson Center
for the Study of Invention and
Innovation, 128-129, 134
Journal of Technology Education, 128
Junior Engineering Technical Society,
93-94, 129

K

K-12, *see* Primary and secondary
education

L

Leadership, 3-4, 9, 12, 16, 26, 59-63,
111-112, 114
Learning by Design, 123
Learning processes, 57-58
Legislation, 62, 111
California energy crisis, 32-36
Carl D. Perkins Vocational
Education Act, 82
educational, 59-62, 82, 84
National Environmental Protection
Act, 38
School to Work Opportunities Act,
84
Lemelson Center for the Study of
Invention and Innovation,
128, 134
Loka Institute, 95, 129
*Longitude: The True Story of a Lone
Genius Who Solved the Greatest
Scientific Problem of His Time*,
118

M

Madison, James, 11
Man-Made World, 77-78
Manufacturing Is Cool!, 124
Massachusetts Curriculum Frameworks, 126
Mass media, 3-4, 7, 14, 20, 90-91, 98,
110, 142
see also Informal education; Internet
Boston Central Artery and Tunnel,
39

computer technology, coverage of,
67, 90-91
fellowship programs, 10, 111-112
news coverage of technology, 66-67,
90-91
Mathematics, 4, 6, 122, 123, 125, 126,
127
characteristics of technologically
literate person, *see*
"characteristics..." under
Technological literacy, general
international test comparisons, 6, 64,
70
state standards, 8, 106
Media influences, *see* Mass media
Medical sciences, *see* Biomedical
sciences
Methodology, 108-110
see also Definitional issues;
Interdisciplinary approaches
assessment of technological literacy,
9, 31, 63-72, 105, 107-110; *see
also* Tests and testing
committee study at hand, *vii-x*, 8,
12, 103
National Science Foundation, 9, 58,
109, 110
Middle School Science and Technology, 79,
124
Minorities, *see* Race/ethnicity
Misconceptions, 5, 50-53
*More Work for Mother: The Ironies of
Household Technology from the
Open Hearth to the Microwave*,
118-119
Multidisciplinary approaches, *see*
Interdisciplinary approaches
Museums, 2, 7, 9, 88-90, 98, 110, 111,
128-129, 141
see also Science and technology
centers

N

Naked City, 48
National Action Council for Minorities
in Engineering, 129
National Aeronautics and Space
Administration, 57, 61, 67,
82, 124, 137, 138, 143, 144
National Assessment of Educational
Progress, 55, 106